ANTI-INFLAMMATORY COOKBOOK

NOURISH YOUR BODY WITH EASY AND HEALING RECIPES - A GUIDE TO INFLAMMATION RELIEF, IMMUNE SYSTEM BOOST, AND DETOXIFICATION, WITH A 30-DAY STRESS-FREE MEAL PLAN

Copyright Notice:

© Grace Garner. All rights reserved. No part of this book may be reproduced, distributed, or transmitted in any form or by any means, without the prior written permission of the author or the publisher, except in the case of brief quotations embodied in critical reviews and certain other noncommercial uses permitted by copyright law.

Liability Disclaimer:

The publisher and author have made every effort to ensure the accuracy and completeness of the information contained in this book. However, neither the publisher nor the author assumes any responsibility for errors, omissions, or contrary interpretation of the subject matter herein. This book is presented "as is" without express or implied warranties. Neither the publisher nor the author shall be liable for any physical, psychological, emotional, financial, or commercial damages, prosecutions, or proceedings incurred as a result of the information provided in this book.

Usage Disclaimer:

This book is intended for informational and entertainment purposes only. The views expressed herein are the personal opinions of the author, and the information provided does not constitute legal, medical, financial or professional advice. Readers are advised to seek appropriate professional consultation before acting upon any information contained in this book.

By reading this book, you acknowledge and agree that you assume the risks associated with any actions you take based on the content of this book and release the author and publisher from any liability.

Acknowledgment of Understanding:

By proceeding beyond this page, the reader acknowledges and agrees to all the terms and conditions set forth within this disclaimer and affirms an understanding of the same.

Severability:

If any provision of this disclaimer is found to be unenforceable, the remaining provisions will continue in full force and effect.

ISBN 979-8-87-896575-0

Table of Contents

Introduction 6
Chapter 01: 6
Understanding the Anti-Inflammatory Diet 7
    Benefits of an Anti-Inflammatory Diet 7
Chapter 02: 9
Practical Tips for Following an Anti-Inflammatory Diet 9
    Foods to Avoid or Limit 9
    Foods To Include 10
    Grocery Shopping Tips 11
    Reading and Understanding Food Labels 12
    How To Make Your Food Delicious? 12
    Tips For Portion Control 13
    Tips for Dining and Social Events 14
    Frequently Asked Questions 14
Chapter 03: Adapting diet for special conditions .. 15
    For Diabetes: 15
    For Heart Health: 15
    For Weight Loss: 15
Chapter 04: Breakfast Recipes 16
    1. Spinach & Egg Scramble 16
    2. Egg & Avocado Toast 16
    3. Healthy Nut Butter Smoothie 16
    4. High Protein Omelet 17
    5. Berry Oatmeal Smoothie 17
    6. Chocolate & Banana Oatmeal 18
    7. Salmon with Scrambled Eggs 18
    8. Fried Egg & Avocado Toast 19
    9. Piña Colada-Inspired Smoothie 19
    10. Strawberry & Tofu Smoothie 19
Chapter 05: Soup Recipes 20
    11. Hearty Lentil Soup with Saffron 20
    12. Vegetable Soup with Pesto 20
    13. Vegetable Soup for Slow Cooker 21
    14. White Bean Pasta Soup 21
    15. Veggie Minestrone Soup 22
    16. Vegetable Soup with Parmesan 23
    17. Slow Cooker Veggie Chili Soup 23
    18. Quick Barley Bean Soup 24
    19. Chicken Ginger & Garlic Soup 24
    20. Veggie-Packed Tofu Soup 25
Chapter 06: Salads & Sides 26
    21. Strawberry Veggie Salad 26
    22. Toasty Turmeric Cauliflower 26
    23. Veggie Tuna Salad 26
    24. Chicken & Mushroom Salad 27
    25. Sweet & Smoky Roasted Broccoli 27
    26. Easy Sauteed Spinach 28
    27. Creamy Kale Salad 28
    28. Creamy White Beans & Avocado Salad 28
    29. Whole Grain Quinoa & Pea Salad 29
    30. Chickpea & Pomegranate Salad 29
Chapter 07: Meat & Poultry 30
    31. Baked Chicken & Vegetables with Romesco Sauce 30
    32. Creamy Chicken One Pot Pasta 30
    33. Quick Beef Curry with Rice 31
    34. Easy Chicken Marsala 31
    35. Ground Beef Pasta 32
    36. Quick & Crispy Chicken Thighs 32
    37. Bacon with Brussels Sprouts 33
    38. Meatballs & Garlic-Lemon Orzo 33
    39. Sweet & Spicy Pork Kebabs 34
    40. Grilled Steak with Salad Dressing 35
Chapter 08: Fish & Seafood 36
    41. Salmon Piccata with Sauce 36

- 42. Quick Crispy Salmon 36
- 43. Simple Blackened Catfish 37
- 44. Seasoned Grilled Red Snapper Fish 37
- 45. Crusted Sweet Scallops 38
- 46. Panko & Pistachio Crusted Halibut 38
- 47. One Pot Shrimp with Spinach 39
- 48. One Pot Shrimp & Broccoli 40
- 49. Mediterranean-Style Cod with Tomatoes.... 40
- 50. Crispy Pan-Fried White Bass 41
- 51. Hearty Shrimp & Fish Stew 41
- 52. Simple Baked Fish Fillets 42
- 53. Calamari with Fresh Herbs Salad 43
- 54. Fish Fillets with Lemon-Dill Sauce 43
- 55. Salmon & Peppercorn Sauce 44

Chapter 09: Vegetarian & Vegan Dishes 45
- 56. Toasted Shishito Peppers 45
- 57. Burrata Pasta with Cherry Tomatoes 45
- 58. Moo-Shu Chinese Style Vegetables 46
- 59. Garlic Pea Shoots Stir Fry 47
- 60. Spicy Broccoli Stir Fry 47
- 61. Peanut Butter Broccoli Stir Fry 48
- 62. Lemon Asparagus Stir Fry 48
- 63. Toasted Zucchini Stir Fry 49
- 64. Broccoli with Tofu Stir Fry 49
- 65. Chicken-Style Seitan Stir Fry 50
- 66. Chinese green beans stir fry 51
- 67. Creamy Brussels Sprouts with Fettuccine.... 51
- 68. Goat Cheese & Beet Pasta 52
- 69. Chickpea Salad with Cranberry & Walnut.... 52
- 70. Pineapple & Tofu Stir Fry 53

Chapter 10: Snack Recipes 55
- 71. English Muffin with Tuna Salad 56
- 72. Crispy Green Lettuce Wraps with Turkey 56
- 73. Healthy & Creamy Pesto Chicken 57
- 74. Black Beans & Veggie Taco Bowl 57
- 75. Healthy Goat Cheese & Arugula Sandwich .. 58
- 76. Creamy Rotisserie Chicken Bowl 58
- 77. Kale & Sun-Dried Tomatoes Snack 58
- 78. Instant Ramen Noodles with Soft-Boiled Egg59
- 79. Falafel & Tzatziki Tabbouleh Bowls 59
- 80. Creamy Cucumber Salad Sandwich 60

Chapter 11: Dessert Recipes 61
- 81. Sweet & Easy Pistachio & Date Bites 61
- 82. Sweet Fig & Honey Yogurt 61
- 83. Strawberry & Chocolate Yogurt Bark 61
- 84. Old-Fashioned Apple Crisp Dessert 62
- 85. Frozen Chocolate Banana Bites 63
- 86. Date & Mango Energy Bites 63
- 87. Banana Flourless Chocolate Chip Muffins.... 64
- 88. Quick Peach & Pistachio Toast 64
- 89. Quick & Fresh Pineapple Ice Cream 65
- 90. Easy Watermelon Sherbet 65

Chapter 12: Sauces, Condiments & Dressing......... 66
- 91. Spinach & Walnut Pesto 66
- 92. Italian Olive Dressing 66
- 93. Homemade Garlic Aioli 66
- 94. Easy & Creamy Chipotle Sauce 67
- 95. Easy White Wine Sauce 67
- 96. Lemon & Garlic Vinaigrette 68
- 97. Sweet Tart Balsamic Marinade 68
- 98. Quick & Easy Cucumber Pickles 68
- 99. Roasted Garlic Parmesan Cream Sauce........ 69
- 100. Homemade Rosemary & Red Wine Marinade 69

Chapter 13: Quick & Easy Meals 70
- 101. Easy Pesto Ravioli 70
- 102. Buttered & Seared Scallops 70
- 103. Quick Black Bean Quesadillas 71
- 104. Stuffed Potatoes & Salsa 71
- 105. Chicken & Strawberry Poppy Seed Salad ... 71
- 106. Butternut Squash Soup with Halloumi 72
- 107. Teriyaki Edamame Stir Fry 72
- 108. Tex-Mex Black Beans & Fajita 73
- 109. Asparagus & Cauliflower Gnocchi 73

110. Stuffed Sweet Potatoes 74

Chapter 14: Meals on a Budget 75

111. Steamed Green Beans 75
112. Brown Rice & Black Beans Bowl 75
113. Stuffed Avocado with Salmon 75
114. Healthy Kale & Banana Smoothie 76
115. Edamame & Beets Salad 76
116. Indian Paneer Saag 77
117. Tuna with Chickpea Salad 77
118. Sweet Potato & Quinoa Chili 78
119. Orange Tofu with Chipotle 79
120. Quick Vegetarian Chili 79
121. Vegetarian Fried Rice 80
122. Vegetables & Hummus Sandwich 80
123. Chickpea Chile Bowl 81
124. One Pot Chicken & Broccoli Pasta 81
125. Chicken with Spinach Skillet 82

Bonus Chapter 1: Mediterranean Diet Dishes 83

126. Chicken Salsa Verd 83
127. Mushroom & Kale Chickpea Pasta 83
128. Quinoa & Chickpea Bowls 84
129. One Pot Spinach & Chicken Sausage 84
130. Salmon Pita Bread Sandwich 85
131. Chickpea Lettuce Wraps with Tahini 85
132. Mediterranean Tuna Spinach Salad 86
133. Mediterranean-Inspired Lunch Box 86
134. Shrimp & Feta Wrap 86
135. Berry & Chia Pudding 87
136. Spinach Ravioli with Artichokes 87
137. One Pot Chicken Pesto Pasta 88
138. Easy Raspberry Muesli 88
139. Vegetables & Lentil Stew 89
140. One Pot Mediterranean Coconut Curry 89

Bonus Chapter 2: Gluten-Free Dishes 91

141. Gluten-free Creamy Broccoli Salad 91
142. Gluten-free Warm Stuffed Potatoes 91
143. Gluten-free Tomato Mussels 92
144. Gluten-free Broccolini with White Beans ... 92
145. Gluten-free Lemon & Basil Chicken 93

Bonus Chapter 3: Air Fryer Dishes 94

146. Scallops with Lemon Herb Sauce 94
147. Sweet Orange Chicken 94
148. Lemony Lamb Chops 95
149. Quick Tangy Zucchini 95
150. Crumbed Chicken Breasts 96

Chapter 18: Meal Planning and Prep 97

Conclusion 102

Measurement Conversion Table 104

Recipe Index (Alphabetical order) 105

Introduction

Are you really tired of fighting the relentless pain and discomfort caused by acute and chronic inflammation? The endless struggle to find a healthy and lasting solution to treat your inflammation can really be overwhelming. I understand the frustration that comes with such a challenge. That is why I want to introduce you to the transformative power of the anti-inflammatory diet – the perfect solution to your inflammation-related woes.

As a seasoned nutritionist, I have personally witnessed the incredible impact of this dietary approach on my clients. Time and again, I have recommended the anti-inflammatory diet to individuals dealing with both acute and chronic inflammation, and the results were simply amazing.

Inspired by the great feedback and the positive transformations I have seen in the lives of many of my clients, I have decided to create this detailed and comprehensive anti-inflammatory diet cookbook. It's not just for those who have inflammation; it's for everyone who is out there for a healthier, nutritious, and wholesome diet.

Inside this cookbook, there is a comprehensive collection of 150 anti-inflammatory recipes that you will find. These recipes are thoughtfully divided into sections to make your meal planning super convenient. Additionally, I have included a 30-day meal plan and a handy grocery list to help you start your journey to a pain-free life without putting much thought into the planning process. With over 1,500 days' worth of meal ideas in your hand, you will always have a flavorsome serving option to go for.

So, let's not wait any further and get started with exploring the incredible benefits of the anti-inflammatory diet.

Ready to transform your health?

Share your excitement and commitment with us! Your initial review can spark a health revolution, encouraging others to join us in wellness. Dive into the journey, and don't forget to grab your special bonuses in the conclusions section. Let's make health our mission, together.

Chapter 01: Understanding the Anti-Inflammatory Diet

Perhaps inflammation is more damaging to health than we all expect it to be. The inflammation that we need to address affects our health in various ways. There are basically two types of inflammations that an individual can experience in his life. The first is acute inflammation, which is a quick and short-term response in which the immune system sends white blood cells to surround and protect against any recent damage to the cell. The symptoms of this inflammation usually go away in a few hours or 2-3 days. The second is chronic inflammation, which is a long-term condition that slowly affects different parts of the body. Numerous factors can lead to chronic inflammation, like autoimmune diseases, extended exposure to irritants, smoking, chronic stress, etc. Since persistent inflammation may increase the risk of a number of diseases, including rheumatoid arthritis, malignancies, cardiovascular disease, periodontitis, and more, chronic inflammation needs a proper fix.

Now, you can either rely on medicinal therapies to treat your inflammation, which always comes with a long list of side effects, or you simply choose a dietary approach and lifestyle that can prevent or treat the chronic inflammation in the body. Such an anti-inflammatory diet lays out a plan to avoid all the food that triggers inflammation and promotes the use of the food that counters inflammation in the body. Refined sugars, carbs, saturated fats, and fried or processed food with preservatives are responsible for exacerbating chronic inflammation in the body, hence they must be avoided. The antioxidants and phytonutrients present in fresh and organic produce are useful in countering inflammation. By studying the inflammatory and anti-inflammatory properties of food products, the proponents of the anti-inflammatory diet set a bunch of guidelines for using a diet as a natural and healthy means to treat chronic inflammation.

Benefits of an Anti-Inflammatory Diet

Though the anti-inflammatory diet is largely responsible for treating the inflammation in the body, the food recommended in this dietary approach makes it even more beneficial. There are several other health advantages that you can harness through this diet:

Inflammation Reduction:

The first and foremost benefit of this diet is to counter inflammation. This approach helps the body get rid of the toxins that may be contributing to the inflammation.

Improves Heart Problems:

Since the diet removes all the trans-fat, processed meals, and bad cholesterol from our food, its secondary benefit is that it can help maintain blood pressure and strengthen blood vessel function, which in turn keeps the heart healthy.

Improves Joint Conditions:

Illnesses like arthritis, joint pain, and stiffness can be reduced with the help of anti-inflammatory food. Antioxidants from leafy vegetables and fresh fruits and omega-3 fatty acids from fish and flaxseeds strengthen joints and lower inflammation-related problems.

Improves Gut Health:

The billions of bacteria that formulate the gut microbiome are significant for a healthy body. The gut microbiome can directly be affected by inflammatory responses, which contribute to several gastrointestinal issues. An anti-inflammatory diet helps promote good gut health.

Increase Brain Functionality:

Anti-inflammatory foods such as fatty fish and berries maintain brain function and help in lowering the risk of Dementia.

Boosts Energy Level:

Fatigue, or low energy, is caused by constant body inflammation. Eating anti-inflammatory food can lower the inflammation as well as increase the energy levels.

Balanced Blood Sugar:

Balanced Blood sugar plays a key role in lowering the risk of diseases. It can be regulated by anti-inflammatory foods in your diet. It is especially suggested to those having diabetes or who are at the risk of developing it.

Stronger Immunity:

Having a stronger immune system can fight harmful infections and other diseases. A diet rich in anti-inflammatory foods contributes to a healthy immune system because they supply important vitamins, minerals, and antioxidants.

Healthy Skin:

Healthy skin needs vitamins, minerals, and antioxidants. An anti-inflammatory diet provides all these things. Anti-inflammatory foods fight oxidative stress and lower the chance of developing skin problems like acne, bacterial infection, and early aging.

Chapter 02: Practical Tips

Since the market is flooded with a variety of food markets, it is hard to look for every other ingredient and read its labels to identify its anti-inflammatory characteristics. Having a general understanding of the items constituting such a diet is quite important. One simple formula to keep in mind for this is to stay close to the naturally grown food items and follow a balanced dietary routine. Saturated fats and complex proteins can elevate the levels of inflammation; therefore, they should be avoided on an anti-inflammatory diet.

Foods to Avoid or Limit

When it comes to any health-oriented diet, the focus should always remain on what to avoid. Here is the list of the ingredients that directly or indirectly contribute to the factors responsible for inflammation.

1. Nightshade Vegetables

The nightshade vegetables belong to a group of plants, Solanaceae, which naturally carry Solanine, the chemical that is capable of aggravating pain, swelling, and arthritis. For this reason alone, the entire family of nightshade vegetables is restricted to the anti-inflammatory diet. Identifying nightshades, among other vegetables, is tricky! Commonly used nightshade vegetables are as follows, and they should all be equally avoided on the anti-inflammatory diet:

- White potatoes
- Eggplant
- Bell peppers
- Cayenne pepper
- Paprika

In potatoes, Solanine is present in trace amounts, which is considered safe, but the green parts of the potatoes may contain Solanine in high amounts, so the experts have disapproved of it along with green potatoes for this diet plan.

2. Processed meats

All food items that are processed, especially meat, are strictly forbidden on this diet. Why so? Because those items are loaded with preservatives and chemical, which can trigger inflammation or exacerbate it.

3. Sugar and sugary drinks

Sugar is the primary stimulant of inflammation. Excessive glucose excites the cells and triggers the immune system to respond aggressively to all metabolic processes in the body. This regressive response may lead to excessive inflammation. Cut down the intake of brown sugar, white sugar, and all sugary items from your diet, and add low-carb sweeteners instead.

4. Trans Fats and Fried Foods

Trans fats are processed and hydrogenated artificially, which makes them even more harmful than naturally existing saturated fats. Food fried in these trans fats is equally health-damaging. Steamed, smoked, and grilled food is a better and safer option for an anti-inflammatory diet.

5. Gluten, White Bread, And Pasta

Refined carbs are as health-damaging as sugar. And gluten can trigger certain allergies, which leads to inflammation. Therefore, food containing gluten should be avoided on this diet plan, such as white bread or pasta. Instead, use nut-based flours like flaxseed meals, almond flour, or coconut flour, and use pasta made out of gluten-free ingredients.

6. Processed Foods & Snacks

Snack food items are not allowed on an anti-inflammatory diet and for all the obvious reasons. These items are made out of all the raw ingredients which aggravate inflammation. It is better to substitute them with a bowl of berries and a fruity smoothie.

Nature Medicine published a study in December 2019 that says that ultra-processed foods' sugars, grains, and excess salt can alter the flora in your gut, harming the gut lining and activating inflammatory genes in cells.

7. Desserts

Since most dessert we consume contain high content of sugars, refined flour, and gluten; all these ingredients are triggers for inflammation. Therefore, they must be avoided. You can always create sugar-free, low-carb desserts at home using the anti-inflammatory recipes.

8. Excess Alcohol

Excessive alcohol, like sugar, can contribute to inflammation. High intake of alcohol can disrupt the natural metabolic processes, which exacerbates the chronic inflammation.

Foods To Include

Have you ever taken antihistamines? What do those medicines do? They instantly relieve the immune system and treat inflammation. The agents responsible for such relief can also be consumed through our food.

1. Dark Leafy Greens:

All leafy and green vegetables contain antioxidants that support the immune system and strengthen it. These vegetables can either be consumed in meals or through regular drinks and beverages. A warming bowl of green soup or a kiwi smoothie, for instance, can be a good option to consume. Leafy greens are so enriched with antioxidants that their contents are extracted for medicinal use. Avoid overcooking to preserve the natural constituents of these vegetables.

2. All Berries

In fruits, berries form that group of food is recommended to all since they contain lots of antioxidants and fewer carbs and calories. Berries are the healthiest of all the fruits recommended on an anti-inflammatory menu. They can be taken in desserts or snacks and in smoothies. When you use berries regularly in your diet, it can really help fight the inflammation.

3. Dark Red Grapes

The dark red grapes contain resveratrol, which is a phytonutrient known for its quality of boosting the immune system, preventing prostate cancer, and relieving inflammation. The red or dark skin grapes are due to the presence of this anti-inflammatory agent. A good consumption of red grapes is therefore highly recommended on this diet.

4. Vegetables

The non-nightshade vegetables that do not carry Solanine are also recommended on this diet. These veggies are nutrient-dense and do not carry any element that could trigger inflammation. Cauliflower, broccoli, mushrooms, yams, and sweet potatoes all are allowed on this diet.

5. Beans and Lentils

Both beans and lentils are high in fiber and antioxidants, which makes them a suitable ingredient for this diet. Kidney beans, chickpeas, brown lentils, and white beans are all good for reducing inflammation.

6. Green Tea

Green tea contains flavonoids, which are another type of phytonutrients and carry antioxidant properties. Green tea brings relief to all sorts of inflammation. It is recommended for regular use to avoid inflammation. It can either be consumed directly or by adding to sugar-free drinks and juices.

7. Olives and Olive Oil

Adding a good number of olives to the diet brings several nutrients and antioxidants to the table. If you cannot consume olives in your diet regularly, then make maximum use of olive oil in your cooking. A drizzle of olive oil to every salad and serving gives them a good boost of phytonutrients.

8. Avocado and Coconut

Both avocado and coconut are extremely soothing in their properties. They carry all such antioxidants, which effectively reduce inflammation. Coconut flesh, water, milk, and cream are all good for this diet.

9. Nuts and Seeds

Nuts and seeds are great for our health and metabolism. They carry essential oils and a concentrated sum of antioxidants. Nuts-based milk is an excellent choice for an anti-inflammatory diet.

10. Seafood

Seafood contains omega-3, along with other essential nutrients. Salmon and sardines are greatly recommended to reduce inflammation.

11. Dark Chocolate

Yes! Sugar-free dark chocolate is a natural reliever of swelling and pain. Chocolate is good at regulating the release of hormones in the body, supporting the immune system, and strengthening it.

12. Spices and Herbs

Turmeric, cinnamon, thyme, rosemary, parsley, oregano, basil, etc., all such spices and herbs contain anti-inflammatory agents in great amounts, so much that turmeric is even used in skin ointments to treat injuries or burns.

Grocery Shopping Tips

It is difficult to remember all the principles of the anti-inflammatory diet every time you cook something. The best technique is to sort things in your pantry or grocery shop according to this dietary approach. Here are some tips that will assist you while doing grocery shopping:

Follow the Dietary Approach

Plan ahead your meals for a week before the grocery shopping day. You can easily do shopping while sticking to the plan and will not make any unnecessary purchases.

Stick to the Perimeter:

You can start your shopping with fresh fruits and vegetables and dairy goods because most stores have these items on the outside aisle racks. Also, these are the first steps towards an anti-inflammatory diet.

Add Nutritious Fats:

Select healthy fats sources such as avocados, olive oil, nuts, and seeds. They can improve your overall health because of the anti-inflammatory qualities they have.

Herbs and Spices:

Experiment with different herbs and spices except for salt and other unhealthy seasonings to give your food flavor. Cinnamon, ginger, garlic, and turmeric is beneficial to lower inflammation.

Preferring Whole Grains:

While purchasing grains, you need to choose brown rice, quinoa, oats, and whole wheat pasta or bread. Avoid foods that claim to be "enriched" and "refined".

Buy Seasonal Foods:

Purchase foods that are easily available in any season as they don't cost much.

Substitutes of Dairy Products:

Choose low-fat or plain types of food while shopping for dairy products. But if you are allergic to dairy products, you can also go for dairy-free items like almond milk, soy milk, or coconut yogurt.

Frozen Foods:

Your first option is to go for fresh fruits and vegetables, but if the first option is not available, then choose other options like frozen or canned.

Purchase in Bulk Amount:

Buy food in bulk that has longer shelf lives, for example, grains, legumes, and nuts, to save time and money.

Reading and Understanding Food Labels

The concept of an anti-inflammatory diet sounds a bit different from the other health-oriented diet plans as it has different objectives to achieve. It has distinct boundaries and clearly defines what food to take and what to avoid based on its chemical properties. The best advice is to constantly monitor food and its effect on your inflammatory condition. So, while buying products from the supermarket, it is also important to read labels and avoid getting any products that may contain unhealthy ingredients.

Evaluate the serving size:

The serving size is written on the top of the nutrition facts label. Compare the different items and select according to the serving size before looking at the other nutrients listed on the label.

Look for added sugar content:

The amount of added sugar is written after the amount of total fat. Since the inflammation can get aggravated by an excessive amount of sugar intake, products carrying lots of sugar must be avoided.

Watch out for Unhealthy fats:

Tran's fats and saturated fats should be avoided because of the inflammation they cause. You must avoid foods that are typically high in saturated fats or those that contain hydrogenated oils. Instead of those fats, select foods that are rich in omega-3 fatty acids and other healthful fats.

Allergens Check:

People have different types of allergies, and inflammation may worsen by eating allergic foods. Read the labels to find out allergens like gluten, dairy, or soy.

Take sodium into account:

Consuming too much sodium might also cause inflammation. Look for foods that have lower amounts of sodium and stay away from those with a lot of salt added.

How To Make Your Food Delicious?

Whenever people think about a healthy diet, they think that their food has to be boring and tasteless, but this is not true. Healthy food can be delicious as well. To improve the flavor of healthy meals, start utilizing herbs, spices, and other natural flavor enhancers. They not only add flavor but also give a large amount of health advantages. You can enjoy the taste of your food while still sticking to the anti-inflammatory diet by including these ingredients in your meals.

Explore Different Spices and Herbs:

There are countless options when it comes to herbs and spices. Garlic and rosemary, ginger and lemon, and cumin and coriander are a few of the frequently used pairings. Try to use fresh herbs. Dried herbs lack the actual flavor. But if they are not available, you can also use dried herbs; just remember to use less of them because they are more potent.

Don't be afraid to experiment with flavors.

You don't have to settle for boring food just because you are eating healthy. There are plenty of ingredients, like turmeric, ginger, and chili peppers, that pack a punch in terms of taste. You can also enhance the flavors naturally by using things like juices, different types of vinegar, and even a touch of honey in addition to herbs and spices.

Boost your meals with dressings and sauces:

Combine olive oil, vinegar, mustard, honey, and herbs to create your salad dressings and sauces. Even the simplest salads can be elevated with these concoctions. Remember to taste your food as you go along and make any adjustments in terms of seasoning. Sometimes, just a pinch of salt or a squeeze of lemon juice can turn a dish into something.

Experimenting with flavors

When it comes to exploring flavors, it is imperative to keep in mind that discovering flavor combinations you enjoy is crucial. By using natural flavor enhancers, you can create nourishing meals that satisfy your taste buds and promote your well-being.

Tips For Portion Control

For a healthier body, one thing is very important, and that is Portion control. To regulate your body weight, keep an eye on calorie consumption, and make sure you are getting the correct amount of nutrients without overdosing your body. The concept of healthy portion control doesn't mean that you stop eating it; you just need to eat in smaller portions or take your hands back from unhealthy food. If you don't know how to stop overeating, then try the following tricks:

Using a decent size plate:

Diet is a mind game, so if you use a big plate, the meal will appear less and will not satisfy your brain; so, take a standard or smaller-sized plate; it will be more satisfying.

Measuring cups:

It is hard to find the perfect serving size. For this, you should use measuring cups if you can. This doesn't mean you buy a certain cup; you can use any cup that you like, such as any teacups, mugs, or containers. It's just an easy approach for you to steadily measure the suitable amount.

Selective use is advised:

The type of food you select to curb your cravings makes a measurable difference. If there is an apple and chocolate cake, what should you choose? Definitely fruit because it is a healthier option than a chocolate cake. A few pieces of chocolate won't fill you up as much as an apple, yet both foods have about the same number of calories.

Avoid being greedy:

Cook a specific amount of food according to the serving size. If you cook large batches of food, then make sure to store the remaining and keep it preserved for another day.

Tips for Dining and Social Events

Social events can challenge diet plans, but with the right strategies, you can enjoy them without compromising your diet. Here are some dining out tips:

1. Choose restaurants that offer a variety of options, such as grilled fish, chicken, and vegetables.
2. Avoid dining at places that primarily serve processed or fried food.
3. If you are unsure about what to order, don't hesitate to ask the server for recommendations.
4. Keep an eye on portion sizes. When eating out, it's easy to overindulge, so be mindful of how much you are consuming.
5. You can bring an acceptable appetizer or side dish if you are unsure of the menu. In this way, you are sure that you'll eat a nutritious, anti-inflammatory meal.
6. If you find a lot of unhealthy food on the menu, then concentrate on consuming the healthier food at the party. You may pile fruit, veggies, and nuts on your plate.
7. Just because something is being provided to you doesn't mean you have to eat it. Saying no to meals that you don't want to consume is OK.

Frequently Asked Questions

What is an anti-inflammatory diet?

It is a dietary approach that is used to counter inflammation in the body and is known as an anti-inflammatory diet.

How does it work?

Anti-inflammatory foods contain phytochemicals, antioxidants, and fiber, which guard against cellular stressors and immune system-induced inflammation. They also support a healthy gut flora and slow down digestion to minimize spikes in blood sugar levels.

Is this diet suitable for everyone?

Most people can benefit from the Anti-Inflammatory Diet because it emphasizes eating complete, full of nutrient foods. Before making any significant dietary changes, it is always advised to speak with a healthcare provider, especially if you have particular medical issues or dietary limitations.

Can an anti-inflammatory diet contribute to the weight loss?

The answer is yes. An anti-inflammatory diet can aid in producing a calorie deficiency and promoting long-term weight loss. This is because it focuses on whole foods, minimizing processed meals, and encouraging portion control. For best results, you should also do regular exercise while following the diet.

What's the best way to start the anti-inflammatory diet?

To kickstart your journey with the anti-inflammatory diet, focus on few things:

- Consume a lot of fresh fruits and veggies.
- Go for whole grains rather than refined ones.
- Pick healthy protein options, including fish, poultry, and legumes.
- Have control over fried, red, processed, and sugary foods and beverages.

How can I understand and read the food labels?

While reading the food labels, focus on the ingredient list to avoid added sugar and other unhealthy ingredients. Choose items with few ingredients and look for whole, raw ingredients. Give attention to the product's nutrient content and serving sizes.

Chapter 03: Adapting diet for special conditions

For Diabetes:

If you are a diabetic who is facing inflammatory issues, then you will have to alter the diet a little to make it suitable for your specific dietary needs.

• Select food items that are low in processed carbs and added sugar.

• Eat more whole grains, fresh fruits, and green vegetables, which are rich in complex carbs. These foods digest more slowly, which keeps the blood sugar levels stable.

• Include protein in each meal. Protein helps in stabilizing blood sugar levels and slowing digestion speed.

• Choose healthy fats like those in almonds, avocados, and olive oil. Healthy fats can increase insulin and

For Heart Health:

If you want your heart to function optimally, then the inflammatory diet is an effective approach to consider. There are certain changes that you will have to consider to meet all your needs:

• Select healthy protein, which includes fish, poultry, and legumes. These are low in cholesterol and saturated fat.

• Lower the amount of processed and red meat. Blood level rises because of saturated fat and cholesterol levels, which are found high in red meat and processed meats.

• Eat a lot of fruits and vegetables. They have lower cholesterol and saturated fat. Fruits and vegetables are also full of minerals like potassium, magnesium, and vitamin C, which are beneficial for the heart.

• Consume healthy fats like those in almonds, avocados, and olive oil. By using healthy fats, inflammation can be reduced, and blood cholesterol levels can rise too.

For Weight Loss:

Yes, it is possible to control your weight or lose a few pounds on this diet if you manage to make certain adjustments in this diet. The goal is to keep the caloric intake controlled and focus on eating healthy meals with essential nutrients:

• Portion control is your friend here! The more you control your portion size, the easier it will get to keep your caloric intake in check. Try to keep your average caloric intake to 2000 calories per day to avoid any weight gain.

• Eat a lot of fruits and vegetables. Fruits and vegetables are high in fiber and low in calories. Fiber can make you feel pleased and full, which may also inspire you to eat less.

• Select whole grains rather than refined ones. If we compare them, whole grains are more nourishing and a rich source of fiber.

• Pick healthy proteins like fish, poultry, and legumes, which are low in calories.

• Limit the use of fried, red, processed items, and sugary foods and beverages. They are the source of bad fats.

Chapter 04: Breakfast Recipes

1. Spinach & Egg Scramble

Prep Time: 10 minutes
Cook Time: 10 minutes
Servings: 1

Ingredients:
- 2 large eggs
- 1 whole-grain bread slice, toasted
- 1 ½ cups baby spinach
- ½ cup fresh raspberries
- 1 teaspoon canola oil
- A pinch kosher salt
- A pinch black pepper

Instructions:
1. Place a small skillet over medium-high flame and heat canola oil.
2. Stir in spinach for 1-2 minutes until it wilts and remove to a plate.
3. Return the pan to the stove, add eggs and stir for 2-3 minutes to make scrambled eggs.
4. Then transfer the spinach to the eggs and season with salt and pepper.
5. Serve the mixture with a toasted bread slice on a plate with raspberries on the side.

Nutrition (Per Serving): Calories: 296 Fat: 16g Carbohydrates: 21g Protein: 18g Fiber: 7g Sugar: 5gSodium: 394mg

Tip: You can replace canola oil with olive oil and raspberries with strawberries in case of unavailability.

2. Egg & Avocado Toast

Prep Time: 5 minutes
Cook Time: 5 minutes
Servings: 1

Ingredients:
- 1 hardboiled egg, chopped
- 1 slice whole wheat toast
- ¼ avocado
- 1 tablespoon celery
- ½ teaspoon lemon juice
- ½ teaspoon hot sauce
- A pinch salt

Instructions:
1. Add avocado, celery, lemon juice, hot sauce, and salt in a small bowl.
2. Add in egg and mash it until a rough paste is formed
3. Spread it on the toast and serve with tea or coffee.

Nutrition (Per Serving): Calories: 230Fat: 14g Carbohydrates: 17g Protein: 11g Fiber: 5g Sugar: 2gSodium: 406mg

Tip: You can replace celery with spinach in case of unavailability.

3. Healthy Nut Butter Smoothie

Prep Time: 5 minutes
Cook Time: 0 minutes
Servings: 1

Ingredients:
- 1 small banana, frozen
- 1 cup almond milk, unsweetened
- 6 ice cubes
- 2 tablespoons almond butter
- 2 tablespoons unflavored protein powder
- ½ teaspoon ground cinnamon
- 1 tablespoon any preferred sweetener, optional

Instructions:
1. Add all the ingredients except ice in a blender.
2. Blend on high until the smoothie becomes smooth and creamy.
3. Then add ice cubes and blend again until smooth.
4. Pour into a glass and serve immediately.

Nutrition (Per Serving): Calories: 402Fat: 22g Carbohydrates: 37g Protein: 19g Fiber: 9g Sugar: 14gSodium: 376mg

Tip: You can experiment and use different flavored protein powders with this recipe if you prefer a more enhanced taste.

4. High Protein Omelet

Prep Time: 10 minutes
Cook Time: 10 minutes
Servings: 1

Ingredients:
- 2 large eggs
- ¼ avocado, sliced
- 1 cup chopped kale
- 1 tablespoon fresh cilantro, chopped
- 1 tablespoon lime juice
- 2 teaspoons extra-virgin olive oil, divided
- 1 teaspoon low-fat milk
- 1 teaspoon sunflower seeds, unsalted
- 2 pinches salt, divided
- A pinch crushed red pepper

Instructions:
1. Place a nonstick skillet over medium flame and heat a tablespoon oil.
2. Take a small bowl and whisk eggs with milk and 2 pinches salt.
3. Pour the egg mixture into the hot pan and cool until the bottom is firm for 1 - 2 minutes
4. Flip the omelet to the other side and cook until set for 1 minute.
5. Remove the egg to a plate and set aside.
6. Add kale to a small bowl and toss with a teaspoon of oil, cilantro, lemon juice, sunflower seeds, and crushed red pepper.
7. Top the omelet with the kale salad and serve immediately.

Nutrition (Per Serving): Calories: 339Fat: 28g Carbohydrates: 9g Protein: 15g Fiber: 4g Sugar: 2gSodium: 446mg

Tip: You can substitute lime juice with fresh lemon juice.

5. Berry Oatmeal Smoothie

Prep Time: 10 minutes
Cook Time: 0 minutes
Servings: 3

Ingredients:
- ½ cup water
- ½ cup small ice cubes
- ½ cup quick-cooking rolled oats
- ½ cup nonfat/light almond milk
- ½ cup frozen unsweetened/fresh pitted dark sweet cherries, thawed a little

- ¾ cup frozen unsweetened/fresh strawberries, thawed a little
- 2 tablespoons almond butter
- 1 tablespoon honey

Instructions:
1. Mix water and oats in a medium bowl and microwave for a minute.
2. Mix in ¼ cup milk and microwave for another 30-50 seconds until the oats are tender.
3. Set the bowl aside to cool for 5 minutes.
4. Then, add the oats mixture in the blender with the remaining ¼ cup milk.
5. Add in the remaining ingredients except ice cubes.
6. Cover the top and blend until smooth, and scrape the sides as needed.
7. Add in ice cubes, cover and blend again till smooth.
8. Pour the smoothie into glasses and garnish with additional fruit on top.

Nutrition (Per Serving): Calories: 121Fat: 4g Carbohydrates: 21g Protein: 3g Fiber: 3g Sugar: 12gSodium: 41mg

Tip: You can double this recipe to make 6 servings.

6. Chocolate & Banana Oatmeal

Prep Time: 5 minutes
Cook Time: 5 minutes
Servings: 1

Ingredients:
- ½ small banana, sliced
- 1 cup water
- ½ cup old-fashioned rolled oats
- 1 tablespoon chocolate-hazelnut spread
- A pinch salt
- A pinch flaky sea salt

Instructions:
1. Place a small saucepan with water and a pinch salt and flaky sea salt over medium-high flame and bring it to a boil.
2. Add in oats, stir and lower the heat to a medium to cook for 5 minutes until the liquid is absorbed.
3. Take off from heat, cover and let it sit for 3 minutes.
4. Dish out the oatmeal in a bowl and garnish with chocolate and banana.

Nutrition (Per Serving): Calories: 295Fat: 9g Carbohydrates: 50g Protein: 7g Fiber: 6g Sugar: 17gSodium: 231mg

Tip: To make overnight oats for a single person, combine 1/2 cup water and oats both with a pinch of salt in a jar or bowl with lid. Seal it close and refrigerate overnight.

7. Salmon with Scrambled Eggs

Prep Time: 10 minutes
Cook Time: 10 minutes
Servings: 1

Ingredients:
- 2 large eggs
- 1 scallion, sliced
- 1-ounce smoked salmon, chopped
- 2 teaspoons low-fat cream cheese
- 1 teaspoon capers, rinsed

Instructions:
1. Place a small nonstick skillet over medium flame and grease with a cooking spray.
2. Take a small bowl and whisk the eggs in it.
3. Mix in salmon, cream cheese, scallion, and capers until well-combined.
4. Pour the mixture into the hot skillet and stir to cook until scrambled, for 3-4 minutes.
5. Serve immediately with tea or coffee.

Nutrition (Per Serving): Calories: 205Fat: 13g Carbohydrates: 2g Protein: 19g Fiber: 1g Sugar: 1gSodium: 404mg

Tip: To make the recipe more flavorful, season with salt and pepper.

8. Fried Egg & Avocado Toast

Prep Time: 10 minutes
Cook Time: 10 minutes
Servings: 1

Ingredients:
- 1 large egg, fried
- ¼ avocado
- 1 slice whole-wheat bread, toasted
- ¼ teaspoon ground pepper powder
- ⅛ teaspoon garlic powder
- 1 tablespoon sliced scallion, optional
- 1 teaspoon Sriracha, optional

Instructions:
1. Add avocado, garlic and pepper powder in a bowl and gently mash.
2. Spread the mixture onto the toasted slice.
3. Top with fried egg and optional ingredients to serve.

Nutrition (Per Serving): Calories: 271Fat: 18g Carbohydrates: 18g Protein: 12g Fiber: 5g Sugar: 2gSodium: 216mg

Tip: If you would like to make the recipe even more filling, add arugula or your favorite salad greens over the avocado with a slice of tomato.

9. Piña Colada-Inspired Smoothie

Prep Time: 10 minutes
Cook Time: 10 minutes
Servings: 1

Ingredients:
- 1 cup pineapple chunks, frozen
- 1 cup baby kale
- ½ cup vanilla coconut milk, unsweetened
- ½ fresh orange juice
- ¼ cup plain or coconut-flavored Greek yogurt

Instructions:
1. Add all the ingredients in the blender.
2. Blend on medium-low speed until mixed.
3. Increase the speed to medium-high until completely smooth.
4. Pour the smoothie into a glass and serve immediately.

Nutrition (Per Serving): Calories: 213Fat: 3g Carbohydrates: 41g Protein: 9g Fiber: 4g Sugar: 17gSodium: 28mg

Tip: You can substitute the coconut milk with coconut water or any nut milk you have.

10. Strawberry & Tofu Smoothie

Prep Time: 10 minutes
Cook Time: 10 minutes
Servings: 2

Ingredients:
- 10 strawberries, frozen
- 1 cup almond milk
- ½ cup silken tofu
- 2 tablespoons swerve sweetener

Instructions:
1. Add all the ingredients in the blender.
2. Blend on medium-high speed for a minute until smooth and frothy.
3. Pour the smoothie into a glass and serve immediately.

Nutrition (Per Serving): Calories: 171Fat: 3g Carbohydrates: 30g Protein: 5g Fiber: 2g Sugar: 24gSodium: 105mg

Tip: You can substitute almond milk with reduced-fat milk if you are lactose-intolerant.

Chapter 05: Soup Recipes

11. Hearty Lentil Soup with Saffron

Prep Time: 20 minutes
Cook Time: 20 minutes
Servings: 8

Ingredients:
- 2 medium carrots, finely-chopped
- 2 celery stalks, finely-chopped
- 5 oz. spinach, roughly-chopped
- 1-pound red lentils, cleaned & washed
- 4 cups low-sodium vegetable/chicken broth
- 1 ½ cup water, plus more if required
- 1 large onion, finely-chopped
- 3 garlic cloves, minced
- 3 tablespoons extra-virgin olive oil
- 1 tablespoon tomato paste
- 1 teaspoon kosher salt
- 1 teaspoon ground pepper
- ½ teaspoon ground cumin
- ¼ teaspoon turmeric powder
- ¼ teaspoon crushed saffron threads
- Plain yogurt, for garnish
- Chopped fresh mint, for garnish

Instructions:
1. Place a large heavy pot over medium flame and heat oil.
2. Add in onion, celery and carrots, give a stir and leave for 6-7 minutes to soften, not brown.
3. Mix in garlic, cumin, tomato paste, saffron and turmeric, and cook for a minute.
4. Next, pour in the broth, water, lentils, spinach and season with salt and pepper.
5. Lower the heat to a simmer and cover the pot with the lid.
6. Stir in between to avoid vegetables from sticking to the bottom.
7. Cook for at least 20 minutes, or until the vegetables and lentils are tender.
8. If the consistency is thick, add more water if needed.
9. Ladle out the soup into bowls and garnish with yogurt and mint to serve.

Nutrition (Per Serving): Calories: 280Fat: 7g Carbohydrates: 42g Protein: 15g Fiber: 8g Sugar: 2gSodium: 364mg

Tip: You can store the soup in the fridge for three days or freeze it for up to 3 months.

12. Vegetable Soup with Pesto

Prep Time: 20 minutes
Cook Time: 20 minutes
Servings: 8

Ingredients:
- 2 medium carrots, chopped
- 2 celery stalks, chopped
- 2 medium zucchinis, chopped
- 4 Roma tomatoes, seeded & chopped
- 1 medium onion, chopped
- 2 garlic cloves, minced
- 2 (15 oz.) cans low-sodium cannellini, rinsed
- 12 oz. fresh green beans, cut into ½ inch pieces
- 8 cups salt-free chicken broth
- 4 cups kale, chopped
- 2 tablespoons extra-virgin olive oil
- 8 teaspoons prepared pesto
- 2 teaspoons red-wine vinegar
- ¾ teaspoon salt
- ½ teaspoon ground pepper

Instructions:
1. Place a large pot over medium-high flame and heat oil.
2. Add in onion, carrot, green beans, celery and garlic, give a stir in between while leaving vegetables for 10 minutes to soften, not brown.
3. Pour in the broth and let it come to a boil.

4. Lower the heat to a simmer and cover the pot with the lid.
5. Stir in between to avoid vegetables from sticking to the bottom.
6. Cook for at least 10 minutes, or until the vegetables are tender.
7. Next, add in the remaining ingredients except pesto.
8. Bring the soup to a simmer by increasing the heat.
9. Cook for 10 minutes more, or until zucchini and kale is soft.
10. Ladle out the soup into bowls and garnish with a teaspoon of pesto on top.

Nutrition (Per Serving): Calories: 225Fat: 8g Carbohydrates: 28g Protein: 13g Fiber: 8g Sugar: 5gSodium: 406mg

Tip: You can substitute chicken broth with low-sodium vegetable broth and cannellini beans with other white beans.

13. Vegetable Soup for Slow Cooker

Prep Time: 35 minutes
Cook Time: 4 hours
Servings: 8

Ingredients:
- 1 medium onion, chopped
- 2 medium carrots, chopped
- 2 celery stalks, chopped
- 2 medium zucchinis, chopped
- 4 Roma tomatoes, seeded & chopped
- 2 garlic cloves, minced
- 12 oz. fresh green beans, cut into ½ inch pieces
- 2 (15 oz.) cans salt-free cannellini beans, rinsed
- 4 cups kale, chopped
- 4 cups low-sodium vegetable broth
- 1 Parmesan rind, optional
- 8 teaspoons prepared pesto

- 2 teaspoons salt
- 2 teaspoons red wine vinegar
- ½ teaspoon ground pepper

Instructions:
1. Add all the ingredients except pesto and vinegar in a 6-quart slow cooker.
2. Close the lid and cook for 6 hours on the low setting, or high for 4 hours.
3. After, discard the Parmesan rind if you have added it.
4. Stir in vinegar and ladle out the soup into bowls.
5. Serve with a teaspoon of pesto on top.

Nutrition (Per Serving): Calories: 175Fat: 4g Carbohydrates: 26g Protein: 10g Fiber: 8g Sugar: 5gSodium: 714mg

Tip: You can substitute vegetable broth with low-sodium chicken broth and cannellini beans with other white beans.

14. White Bean Pasta Soup

Prep Time: 15 minutes
Cook Time: 15 minutes
Servings: 6

Ingredients:
- 1 (28 oz.) can salt-free diced tomatoes
- 1 (15 oz.) can low-sodium cannellini beans, rinsed
- 8 oz. small elbow whole wheat pasta
- 2 garlic cloves, minced
- 2 cups low-sodium chicken broth/vegetable broth
- 1 ½ cups frozen cut-leaf spinach
- 1 ½ cups frozen Mirepoix (diced onion, celery & carrot)
- 4 tablespoons Parmesan cheese, low-fat, low-fat, grated
- 1 tablespoon extra-virgin olive oil
- 1 teaspoon salt

- 1 teaspoon Italian seasoning
- ¼ teaspoon ground pepper
- ¼ teaspoon crushed red pepper

Instructions:
1. Place a large pot over medium heat and heat oil.
2. Stir in Mirepoix and cook for 3 minutes or until softened.
3. Next, add garlic, salt, Italian seasoning, crushed red pepper, and ground pepper.
4. Stir to mix well for a minute and until fragrant.
5. Add in tomatoes, beans, and broth and let it come to a boil.
6. Lower heat to a simmer and cover with the lid to cook for 10 minutes.
7. Stir in between until the tomatoes start to soften.
8. Meanwhile, place a large saucepan with water and let it boil on high heat.
9. Add pasta in the boiling water and cook according to the package directions.
10. Mix spinach in the soup and stir in pasta in the soup after draining the water.
11. Ladle out the soup into bowls and top with Parmesan cheese, low-fat, low-fat, to serve.

Nutrition (Per Serving): Calories: 277Fat: 5g Carbohydrates: 48g Protein: 12g Fiber: 9g Sugar: 7gSodium: 576mg

Tip: You can keep the pasta separate and only add it in soup whenever you serve the soup to avoid the pasta from become soggy. It's more preferable to use fresh ingredients if you would like to cook from scratch.

15. Veggie Minestrone Soup

Prep Time: 25 minutes
Cook Time: 10 minutes
Servings: 6

Ingredients:
- 1 large celery stalk, halved-lengthwise & sliced
- 1 medium summer squash, halved-lengthwise & sliced
- 1 medium onion, chopped
- 1 medium carrot, chopped
- 2 large garlic cloves, minced
- 1 (15 oz.) can kidney/cannellini beans, rinsed
- 1 (14 oz.) can salt-free diced tomatoes
- 6 cups low-sodium vegetable broth
- 4 cups kale, chopped
- 1 ½ cups whole wheat fusilli
- 2 tablespoons extra-virgin olive oil
- 1 tablespoon red wine vinegar
- 1 teaspoon Italian seasoning
- ½ teaspoon ground pepper
- ¼ teaspoon salt

Instructions:
1. Place a large pot over medium flame and heat oil.
2. Add in celery, onion, and carrot to cook for 3 minutes and stir until it softens.
3. Next, add garlic, Italian seasoning, salt and pepper and stir for a minute.
4. Pour in broth, add tomatoes, and let it come to a boil.
5. Add squash, kale, and stir in pasta.
6. Bring it to a boil once again and lower heat to a consistent simmer.
7. Stir occasionally and cook for 10 minutes or until the vegetables and pasta become tender.
8. Remove the pot from heat and mix in beans and vinegar.
9. Ladle out the soup into bowls and serve immediately.

Nutrition (Per Serving): Calories: 232Fat: 6g Carbohydrates: 38g Protein: 8g Fiber: 8g Sugar: 7gSodium: 279mg

Tip: You can use a similar type of whole wheat fusilli pasta if it's not available.

16. Vegetable Soup with Parmesan

Prep Time: 25 minutes
Cook Time: 25 minutes
Servings: 4

Ingredients:
- 4 cups low-sodium vegetable/chicken broth
- 4 cups dark leafy greens with stems, like kale/chard, chopped
- 3 cups cubed hard vegetables, carrot/sweet potato/winter squash/turnip
- 2 cups green cabbage, thinly-sliced
- 1 cup cubed soft vegetables, zucchini, halved green beans, broccoli or cauliflower florets or corn kernels
- ½ cup onion, chopped
- 3 garlic cloves, minced
- 3 tablespoons extra-virgin olive oil
- 1 ½ tablespoons tomato paste
- 2 teaspoons sherry vinegar
- 1 teaspoon ground cumin
- 1 teaspoon smoked paprika
- 1 teaspoon dried thyme
- ¾ teaspoon salt
- ½ teaspoon ground pepper

Instructions:
1. Place a large pot over medium flame and heat oil.
2. Add in onions, stir and let soften for 2 minutes.
3. Stir in cumin, garlic, thyme and paprika for a half a second or until fragrant.
4. Stir in hard vegetables and cook for 2 minutes or until softened.
5. Stir in soft vegetables and mix well.
6. Pour in broth, tomato paste and season with salt and pepper.
7. Let it come to a boil on high heat and lower the heat to a consistent simmer.
8. Cover the pot partially and cook the vegetables for 15-20 minutes or until soft.
9. Remove the pot from heat and stir in the vinegar.
10. Ladle out the soup into bowls and serve immediately.

Nutrition (Per Serving): Calories: 211Fat: 11g Carbohydrates: 26g Protein: 4g Fiber: 6g Sugar: 7gSodium: 513mg

Tip: You can store the soup in the refrigerator for upto three days. If you don't have sherry wine, use red wine vinegar instead.

17. Slow Cooker Veggie Chili Soup

Prep Time: 20 minutes
Cook Time: 6 hours
Servings: 8

Ingredients:
- 2 (14.5 oz.) cans salt-free diced fire-roasted tomatoes, undrained
- 1 (15 oz.) can salt-free black beans, rinsed
- 4 cups sweet potatoes, cubed & with peel
- 2 ½ cups salt-free vegetable broth
- 2 cups yellow onion, chopped
- 1 cup loosely-packed fresh cilantro, chopped
- ¼ cup salt-free tomato paste
- 5 garlic cloves, minced
- 1 ½ tablespoons chili powder
- 1 tablespoon fresh lime juice
- 1 ½ teaspoons ground cumin
- ¾ teaspoon salt
- ½ teaspoon ground pepper
- 1 (8 oz.) package shredded Cheddar cheese, for garnish

Instructions:
1. Take a 6-quart slow cooker and add tomatoes, sweet potatoes, beans, broth, onion, tomato paste, cumin, chili powder, garlic, salt and pepper inside.

2. Close the lid and cook for 6 hours on low or until the vegetables become tender.
3. Mix in cilantro and lemon juice.
4. Ladle out the soup into bowls and serve with a sprinkle of cheese on top.

Nutrition (Per Serving): Calories: 174Fat: 1g Carbohydrates: 35g Protein: 6g Fiber: 8g Sugar: 11gSodium: 399mg

Tip: Keeping the peel of the sweet potatoes on increases the fiber ratio of the soup, and is more filling. However, you can remove the peel according to your personal preference.

18. Quick Barley Bean Soup

Prep Time: 15 minutes
Cook Time: 30 minutes
Servings: 4

Ingredients:
- 1 (15 oz.) can white beans, rinsed
- 1 (14 oz.) can fire-roasted tomatoes, diced
- 1 large onion, chopped
- 1 medium fennel bulb, cored & chopped
- 5 garlic cloves, minced
- 6 cups package baby spinach
- 6 cups low-sodium vegetable broth
- ¾ cup quick-cooking barley
- ¼ cup Parmesan cheese, low-fat, low-fat, grated
- 4 teaspoons extra-virgin olive oil
- 1 teaspoon dried basil
- ¼ teaspoon ground pepper

Instructions:
1. Place a Dutch oven or large cast-iron pot over medium flame and heat oil.
2. Stir in garlic, onion, fennel, and basil.
3. Cook for 6-8 minutes until it starts to brown and becomes tender.
4. Add ½ cup beans to the pot after mashing it and add the other half whole.

5. Pour in the broth and stir in tomatoes and barley into the pot.
6. Let it come to a boil over high heat and lower the heat to a simmer to medium heat.
7. Stir occasionally and cook for 15 minutes or until the barley becomes soft.
8. Next, stir in spinach and cook until wilted for a minute.
9. Remove the pot from the heat and ladle out the soup into bowl.
10. Sprinkle cheese on top and season with pepper to serve.

Nutrition (Per Serving): Calories: 333Fat: 8g Carbohydrates: 55g Protein: 13g Fiber: 12g Sugar: 11gSodium: 619mg

Tip: You can store the soup in the fridge for up to 3 days or freeze it for over 3 months.

19. Chicken Ginger & Garlic Soup

Prep Time: 20 minutes
Cook Time: 25 minutes
Servings: 4

Ingredients:
- 1-pound boneless, skinless chicken thighs, trimmed & cut-into-½-inch-pieces
- 4 cups low-sodium chicken broth
- 2 cups malunggay leaves, chopped
- 1 ½ cups peeled & cubed green papaya
- ½ cup yellow onion, chopped
- ¼ cup fresh ginger, thinly-sliced
- 6 garlic cloves, minced
- 3 tablespoons canola/avocado oil
- 1 tablespoon fish sauce
- ¼ teaspoon salt
- ¼ teaspoon ground black pepper

Instructions:
1. Place a large pot over medium flame and heat oil.
2. Add garlic, onions and ginger, stir and cook for 3 minutes or until translucent.

3. Add chicken and broth and stir gently for 5 minutes until the chicken changes
4. color from pink to white.
5. Add in malunggay leaves, papaya, fish sauce, salt, and pepper.
6. Give a stir and let it simmer for 5 minutes or until the vegetables become tender.
7. Remove the pot from heat and ladle out the soup to serve immediately.

Nutrition (Per Serving): Calories: 344Fat: 21g Carbohydrates: 14g Protein: 27g Fiber: 2g Sugar: 6gSodium: 663mg

Tip: You can use bok choy leaves if malunggay leaves are not available. And use chayote instead of green papaya.

20. Veggie-Packed Tofu Soup

Prep Time: 20 minutes
Cook Time: 25 minutes
Servings: 4

Ingredients:
- 1 (14.5 oz.) can salt-free diced tomatoes with basil, garlic and oregano, undrained
- 1 (12 oz.) package extra-firm, tub-style tofu, drained & cut-into-¾-inch-cubes
- 3 cups fresh button mushrooms, sliced
- 2 cups low-sodium chicken broth
- ½ cup fresh/frozen peas, thawed
- ½ cup asparagus, 1-inch pieces
- ½ cup roasted red sweet pepper, chopped
- ⅓ cup oil-packed dried tomatoes, drained & finely-chopped
- ¼ cup green olives, sliced
- 2 tablespoons olive oil
- 1 teaspoon dried Italian seasoning, crushed
- 1 pinch Parmesan cheese, low-fat, shredded
- Nonstick cooking spray, as needed

Instructions:
1. Place a 5–6-quart Dutch oven over medium-high flame and grease with nonstick cooking spray.
2. But before that, add tofu in a resealable plastic bag placed in a shallow bowl.
3. Add oil and Italian seasoning in the tofu bag and seal the bag closed.
4. Turn the bag to coat the tofu and refrigerate for 2 - 4 hours.
5. After, when the Dutch oven is hot, add undrained marinated tofu in it and cook for 5-6 minutes until the tofu is browned and flip only once.
6. Pour broth in and add canned tomatoes, and let it come to a boil.
7. Next, stir in mushrooms, asparagus, and peas, and lower heat to a simmer.
8. Cook the vegetables for 5 minutes or until tender.
9. Add in dried tomatoes, olives, and sweet pepper, and give a stir.
10. Remove from heat and ladle out the soup into bowls.
11. Serve with shredded cheese on top!

Nutrition (Per Serving): Calories: 259Fat: 15g Carbohydrates: 19g Protein: 16g Fiber: 10g Sugar: 11gSodium: 574mg

Tip: If frozen peas are not available, you can add canned ones. Also, if the soup is not soupy enough, add another can of chicken broth for your personal preference.

Chapter 06: Salads & Sides

21. Strawberry Veggie Salad

Prep Time: 5 minutes
Cook Time: 5 minutes
Servings: 1

Ingredients:
- ¼ medium avocado, diced
- 3 cups baby spinach
- ½ cup strawberries, sliced
- 2 tablespoons vinaigrette
- 2 tablespoons toasted walnut pieces
- 1 tablespoon red onion, finely-chopped

Instructions:
1. Toss together onion, spinach, and strawberries in a bowl.
2. Drizzle the vinaigrette on top and toss once again to combine well.
3. Sprinkle avocado and walnuts on top and serve immediately.

Nutrition (Per Serving): Calories: 296Fat: 18g Carbohydrates: 27g Protein: 8g Fiber: 10g Sugar: 11gSodium: 195mg

Tip: Try Annie's Light Raspberry Vinaigrette or Maple Grove Fat Free Poppyseed for dressing.

22. Toasty Turmeric Cauliflower

Prep Time: 10 minutes
Cook Time: 20 minutes
Servings: 5

Ingredients:
- 8 cups cauliflower florets
- 2 large garlic cloves, minced
- 3 tablespoons extra-virgin olive oil
- 2 teaspoons lemon juice
- 1 ½ teaspoons ground turmeric
- ½ teaspoon salt
- ½ teaspoon ground cumin
- ½ teaspoon ground pepper

Instructions:
1. Start by preheating the oven at 425°F.
2. Mix oil, cumin, garlic, turmeric, salt and pepper in a large bowl.
3. Add cauliflower in this dressing and toss to coat.
4. Take a large rimmed baking sheet and transfer the cauliflower onto it.
5. Roast, changing sides once, for 15-25 minutes until browned and tender.
6. Drizzle lemon juice over the cauliflower before serving.

Nutrition (Per Serving): Calories: 124Fat: 9g Carbohydrates: 10g Protein: 4g Fiber: 4g Sugar: 3gSodium: 285mg

Tip: If you like more tang, squeeze one lemon in the dressing as well and drizzle an additional one over the finished dish.

23. Veggie Tuna Salad

Prep Time: 10 minutes
Cook Time: 10 minutes
Servings: 1

Ingredients:
- ½ (5 oz.) can water-packed tuna
- 2 cups baby spinach
- ¼ cup avocado, diced
- ¼ cup cherry tomatoes, halved
- 1 ½ tablespoons poppy seed dressing
- 1 tablespoon red onion, diced
- 1 tablespoon extra-virgin olive oil
- 1 tablespoon sunflower seeds

Instructions:

1. Add avocado, tuna, tomatoes, onion, poppy seed dressing and oil in a bowl.
2. Toss well together and serve this over spinach leaves with a sprinkling of sunflower seeds on top.

Nutrition (Per Serving): Calories: 432Fat: 32g Carbohydrates: 17g Protein: 20g Fiber: 7g Sugar: 8gSodium: 551mg

Tip: If poppy seed dressing is unavailable, you can use French dressing instead.

24. Chicken & Mushroom Salad

Prep Time: 10 minutes
Cook Time: 10 minutes
Servings: 1

Ingredients:
- 12 oz. cooked chicken, shredded
- 4 cups fresh cremini mushrooms, shaved
- 4 cups packed baby arugula
- 4 cups Brussels sprouts, shaved
- 1 cup celery, thinly-diagonally-sliced
- 1 cup Parmesan cheese, low-fat, shaved
- 6 tablespoons olive oil
- 3 tablespoons red-wine vinegar
- 1 ½ tablespoons shallot, minced
- 1 tablespoon Dijon mustard
- 2 teaspoons fresh thyme, chopped
- ½ teaspoon ground pepper

Instructions:
1. Mix oil, vinegar, mustard, shallot, thyme, and pepper in a bowl.
2. Add in chicken, Brussels sprouts, arugula, celery, and mushrooms in the bowl.
3. Toss well together and sprinkle Parmesan cheese, low-fat, low-fat, before serving.

Nutrition (Per Serving): Calories: 384Fat: 31g Carbohydrates: 15g Protein: 24g Fiber: 5g Sugar: 6gSodium: 533mg

Tip: If you'd like a more vegan version, you can skip the chicken.

25. Sweet & Smoky Roasted Broccoli

Prep Time: 15 minutes
Cook Time: 15 minutes
Servings: 6

Ingredients:
- 1 pound broccoli florets
- 3 tablespoons extra-virgin olive oil
- 1 tablespoon fresh lemon/lime juice
- 4 teaspoons honey
- 2 teaspoons canned chipotle in adobo, minced
- 1 teaspoon garlic powder
- ¼ teaspoon salt

Instructions:
1. Start by preheating the oven at 425 degrees F.
2. Take a large rimmed baking sheet and grease it with cooking spray.
3. Mix oil, lemon juice, honey, chipotle, garlic powder, and salt in a large bowl.
4. Add in the broccoli florets and toss well and transfer the broccoli to the baking sheet.
5. Roast for 12-15 minutes, or until tender and browned, flipping once in between. Serve as a side dish with a main dish.

Nutrition (Per Serving): Calories: 104Fat: 7g Carbohydrates: 9g Protein: 3g Fiber: 2g Sugar: 5gSodium: 132mg

Tip: Serve this with grilled fish or roasted chicken to enhance the flavor of the main dish even more.

26. Easy Sauteed Spinach

Prep Time: 10 minutes
Cook Time: 10 minutes
Servings: 4

Ingredients:
- 1-pound frozen cut-leaf spinach
- ¼ cup currants
- 1 small onion, chopped
- 1 garlic clove, minced
- 2 tablespoons pine nuts, toasted
- 2 teaspoons extra-virgin olive oil
- Balsamic vinegar, as needed
- Salt & freshly ground pepper, as needed

Instructions:
1. Place a skillet over medium flame and heat oil.
2. Stir in garlic and onion until it starts to soften.
3. Stir in spinach and cook until wilted.
4. Add in pine nuts, currants, a drizzle of balsamic vinegar, salt and pepper to taste.
5. Stir and serve as a side dish.

Nutrition (Per Serving): Calories: 117Fat: 6g Carbohydrates: 14g Protein: 5g Fiber: 4g Sugar: 8gSodium: 122mg

Tip: If balsamic vinegar is not available, use simple vinegar instead.

27. Creamy Kale Salad

Prep Time: 10 minutes
Cook Time: 10 minutes
Servings: 4

Ingredients:
- 8 oz. trimmed Brussels sprouts
- 4 cups kale, any tough stems removed, roughly-chopped
- 2 cups peeled broccoli stems/broccoli slaw, matchstick-cut
- ½ cup radicchio, sliced
- ¼ cup mayonnaise
- 3 tablespoons dried cranberries
- 3 tablespoons toasted pepitas
- 2 tablespoons cider vinegar
- 1 tablespoon extra-virgin olive oil
- 1 teaspoon poppy seeds
- 1 teaspoon sugar/honey
- ¼ teaspoon salt
- ¼ teaspoon ground pepper

Instructions:
1. Mix oil, vinegar, mayonnaise, sugar/honey, poppy seeds, salt and pepper in a bowl.
2. Add in broccoli stems or slaw, kale, radicchio, cranberries, broccoli sprouts, and pepitas.
3. Toss well to coat and serve with a main dish.

Nutrition (Per Serving): Calories: 158Fat: 12g Carbohydrates: 11g Protein: 4g Fiber: 3g Sugar: 4gSodium: 181mg

Tip: If radicchio is not available, simply use red cabbage.

28. Creamy White Beans & Avocado Salad

Prep Time: 10 minutes
Cook Time: 10 minutes
Servings: 1

Ingredients:
- ½ avocado, diced
- 2 cups mixed salad greens
- ¾ cup veggies of your preference
- ⅓ cup canned white beans, rinsed & drained
- 1 tablespoon red-wine vinegar
- 2 teaspoons extra-virgin olive oil
- ¼ teaspoon kosher salt
- Freshly ground pepper, as needed

Instructions:

1. Add beans, avocado, mixed greens, and your preferred veggies in a bowl to combine.
2. Drizzle vinegar and olive oil on top and toss well to coat, while seasoning with salt and pepper.
3. Serve as a side dish with a main dish.

Nutrition (Per Serving): Calories: 360 Fat: 25g Carbohydrates: 30g Protein: 10g Fiber: 13g Sugar: 3g Sodium: 321mg

29. Whole Grain Quinoa & Pea Salad

Prep Time: 10 minutes
Cook Time: 10 minutes
Servings: 6

Ingredients:
- 1 (10 oz.) package frozen peas
- 2 cups cooked quinoa
- ¼ cup crumbled goat cheese
- 1 shallot, chopped
- 1 lemon zest
- 1 tablespoon extra-virgin olive oil
- ½ teaspoon ground pepper
- ¾ teaspoon salt

Instructions:
1. Place a large skillet over medium flame and heat oil.
2. Cook shallot while stirring for 2 minutes until softened.
3. Add in peas and quinoa, and stir occasionally to cook for 5 minutes until hot.
4. Lastly, stir in zest, cheese, salt and pepper.
5. Serve as a salad with a main dish or eat as it is.

Nutrition (Per Serving): Calories: 148 Fat: 5g Carbohydrates: 21g Protein: 6g Fiber: 4g Sugar: 3g Sodium: 369mg

Tip: To give the salad a stronger flavor, you can add garlic and ginger to the onions while sauteing.

30. Chickpea & Pomegranate Salad

Prep Time: 10 minutes
Cook Time: 10 minutes
Servings: 6

Ingredients:
- 1 (15 oz.) can low-sodium chickpeas, rinsed
- 8 oz. bite-size broccoli florets
- ½ cup pomegranate seeds
- ⅓ cup whole-milk plain yogurt
- ¼ cup red onion, thinly-sliced
- 2 tablespoons extra-virgin olive oil
- 2 tablespoons tahini
- 1 tablespoon lemon juice
- ½ teaspoon ground pepper
- ½ teaspoon ground cumin
- ¾ teaspoon salt, divided

Instructions:
1. Place a small skillet over medium flame, make sure it's dry.
2. Meanwhile, add onion to a bowl of cold water for 10 minutes to soak. Drain after!
3. Next, toast cumin on the hot skillet for 1-2 minutes until fragrant and remove to a large bowl.
4. Add tahini, yogurt, oil, lemon juice, half teaspoon salt and pepper to the cumin bowl.
5. Whisk this all together until smooth and add in chickpeas, broccoli, onion, and pomegranate seeds.
6. Toss well to combine and let it sit for 10 minutes.
7. Toss again after adding the remaining ¼ tsp of salt.

Nutrition (Per Serving): Calories: 162 Fat: 9g Carbohydrates: 16g Protein: 6g Fiber: 4g Sugar: 4g Sodium: 344mg

Tip: You can refrigerate this for up to 1 day.

Chapter 07: Meat & Poultry

31. Baked Chicken & Vegetables with Romesco Sauce

Prep Time: 20 minutes
Cook Time: 30 minutes
Servings: 4

Ingredients:
- 4 bone-in chicken thighs, skinless & fat-trimmed
- 2 large Yukon Gold potatoes, cubed
- 1 (7 oz.) jar roasted red peppers, rinsed
- 4 cups broccoli florets
- ¼ cup slivered almonds
- 4 tablespoons extra-virgin olive oil, divided
- 1 small garlic clove, crushed
- 1 teaspoon paprika
- 1 teaspoon ground pepper, divided
- ½ teaspoon salt, divided
- ½ teaspoon ground cumin
- ¼ teaspoon crushed red pepper
- Chopped fresh cilantro, for garnish

Instructions:
1. Start by preheating the oven at 450 degrees F.
2. Take a medium bowl and toss potatoes in it with a teaspoon of oil, ⅛ teaspoon salt, and ¼ teaspoon ground pepper.
3. Transfer them to one side of a large baking rimmed sheet.
4. Take another bowl and toss chicken with a tablespoon oil, ⅛ teaspoon salt, and ¼ teaspoon ground pepper.
5. Transfer the chicken to the empty place of the baking sheet and bake for 15 minutes.
6. Meanwhile, add broccoli to a bowl with 2 teaspoons oil, ¼ teaspoon pepper, and ⅛ teaspoon salt.
7. Toss well and once the potatoes and chicken have roasted after 10 minutes, transfer the broccoli onto the potatoes side of the baking sheet.
8. Combine the vegetables together and move forward with the roasting until the chicken and vegetables are tender for 15 minutes more.
9. Meanwhile, add the remaining 2 tablespoons oil, ⅛ teaspoon salt, and ¼ teaspoon ground pepper with roasted peppers, crushed red pepper, paprika, cumin, garlic, and almonds into a mini food processor.
10. Pulse until everything is smooth like a sauce.
11. Serve this sauce with roasted chicken and vegetables, and sprinkle cilantro on top!

Nutrition (Per Serving): Calories: 499Fat: 27g Carbohydrates: 30g Protein: 33g Fiber: 5g Sugar: 2gSodium: 665mg

Tip: If you don't prefer chicken thighs or their unavailable, you can use chicken tenders instead.

32. Creamy Chicken One Pot Pasta

Prep Time: 35 minutes
Cook Time: 5 minutes
Servings: 5

Ingredients:
- 1-pound boneless, skinless chicken thighs
- 8 oz. whole-wheat linguine/spaghetti
- 4 cups mushrooms, sliced
- 4 cups water
- 2 cups Brussels sprouts, sliced
- 1 medium onion, chopped
- 4 garlic cloves, thinly-sliced
- 2 tablespoons fresh chives, chopped
- 2 tablespoons Boursin cheese
- 1 ¼ teaspoons dried thyme
- ¾ teaspoon dried rosemary

- ¾ teaspoon salt

Instructions:
1. Place a large pot of water and put it over high heat.
2. Add pasta, chicken, Brussels sprouts, mushrooms, onion, garlic, cheese, rosemary, thyme, and salt into the water.
3. Give it all a stir and bring to a boil.
4. Stir occasionally until the water evaporates in 10-15 minutes.
5. Remove the pot from heat and let it rest for a few minutes.
6. Serve the pasta onto plates with a sprinkling of extra chives on top.

Nutrition (Per Serving): Calories: 353Fat: 10g Carbohydrates: 42g Protein: 27g Fiber: 8g Sugar: 4gSodium: 461mg

Tip: If Boursin cheese is unavailable, you can use low fat cream cheese instead. Also, for more flavor, you can use low-sodium chicken broth instead of water.

33. Quick Beef Curry with Rice

Prep Time: 10 minutes
Cook Time: 10 minutes
Servings: 4

Ingredients:
- 12 oz. beef tenderloin, thinly-sliced
- 1 (13.5 oz.) can light coconut milk
- 2 cups hot cooked brown basmati rice
- 1 cup torn fresh basil leaves
- 1 cup sliced onion
- 2 tablespoons fresh lime juice
- 4 teaspoons red curry paste
- 2 teaspoons dark brown sugar
- 2 teaspoons fish sauce
- ½ teaspoon kosher salt
- ¼ teaspoon crushed red pepper
- 4 lime wedges, for garnish

Instructions:
1. Place a large skillet over medium flame.
2. Use a spoon to spoon out coconut cream—the thick layer of top of the coconut milk can.
3. Add in the curry paste by stirring and bring this all to a boil on medium-high heat.
4. Next, pour in the remaining coconut milk and mix in fish sauce, sugar, and red pepper.
5. Bring it to a boil and cook it for 2 minutes by continuously stirring before adding onion.
6. Lower heat to medium and let it simmer for 4 minutes.
7. Stir in beef next and cook for 3 minutes until tender.
8. Remove the skillet from heat and mix in lemon juice, basil, and salt.
9. Serve the beef curry with rice and lime wedges on top.

Nutrition (Per Serving): Calories: 334Fat: 11g Carbohydrates: 36g Protein: 24g Fiber: 8g Sugar: 2gSodium: 645mg

Tip: Don't shake the coconut milk can before opening, you should keep the thick layer of coconut cream separate which is needed in the recipe.

34. Easy Chicken Marsala

Prep Time: 10 minutes
Cook Time: 10 minutes
Servings: 4

Ingredients:
- 4 (4 oz.) chicken breast cutlets, skinless & boneless
- 1 (8 oz.) package button mushrooms, pre-sliced
- ⅔ cup unsalted chicken stock
- ⅔ cup Marsala wine
- 4 thyme sprigs
- 2 ½ tablespoons unsalted butter
- 2 tablespoons olive oil, divided

- 1 tablespoon all-purpose flour
- 1 tablespoon chopped fresh thyme, optional
- ¾ teaspoon black pepper, divided
- ½ teaspoon kosher salt, divided

Instructions:
1. Place a large skillet over medium heat and heat a tablespoon of oil.
2. Season chicken with salt and pepper, and add it to the skillet.
3. Cook each side for 4 minutes or until done.
4. Remove the chicken from the pan and add the remaining oil to the skillet.
5. Stir in mushrooms and thyme to cook for 6 minutes until browned.
6. Stir in flour and continue mixing for a minute.
7. Pour stock and wine in the skillet and let it come to a boil on high heat.
8. Thicken it for 2-3 minutes and remove from the heat.
9. Stir in the butter and the remaining salt and pepper.
10. Add the chicken in the skillet and flip to coat properly.
11. Discard the thyme sprigs before serving.
12. Serve with chopped thyme sprinkled on top!

Nutrition (Per Serving): Calories: 344Fat: 17g Carbohydrates: 9g Protein: 27g Fiber: 1g Sugar: 7gSodium: 567mg

Tip: You can pair this saucy chicken with thin spaghetti or rice.

35. Ground Beef Pasta

Prep Time: 35 minutes
Cook Time: 15 minutes
Servings: 4

Ingredients:
- 1 pound 90% lean ground beef
- 1 (15 oz.) can no-salt-added tomato sauce
- 8 oz. whole-wheat rotini or fusilli
- 8 oz. mushrooms, finely-chopped
- 1 cup water
- ½ cup onion, diced
- ½ cup extra-sharp Cheddar cheese, shredded
- 1 tablespoon extra-virgin olive oil
- 1 tablespoon Worcestershire sauce
- 1 teaspoon Italian seasoning
- ¾ teaspoon salt
- ½ teaspoon garlic powder
- ¼ cup chopped fresh basil, for garnish

Instructions:
1. Place a large skillet over medium flame and heat oil.
2. Stir occasionally and cook mushrooms, beef, and onion for 8-10 minutes until the beef is no longer pink and the liquid of the mushrooms has evaporated.
3. Add and stir in water, tomato sauce, Worcestershire sauce, Italian seasoning, salt and garlic powder.
4. Add in pasta and let it come to a boil on high flame.
5. Close the lid and lower heat to cook until the pasta is soft for 16-18 minutes and most of the liquid has been absorbed by the pasta.
6. Sprinkle cheese and cover for it to melt and then sprinkle basil on top before serving.

Nutrition (Per Serving): Calories: 582Fat: 21g Carbohydrates: 55g Protein: 44g Fiber: 8g Sugar: 5gSodium: 691mg

Tip: This recipe is great to sneak in some veggies that are leftover or when your family doesn't eat vegetables on their own.

36. Quick & Crispy Chicken Thighs

Prep Time: 15 minutes
Cook Time: 10 minutes
Servings: 4

Ingredients:

- 6 (6 oz.) bone-in & skin-on chicken thighs, extra-fat-trimmed
- 1 tablespoon canola oil
- 1 teaspoon paprika
- 1 teaspoon kosher salt
- 1 teaspoon freshly-ground black pepper

Instructions:
1. Start by preheating the oven at 500-degree F.
2. Meanwhile, put chicken thighs skin side up on a cutting board and put plastic wrap over them.
3. Use a chicken mallet or a small heavy cast-iron or skillet pan to pound chicken to ¾ inch thickness.
4. Take a paper towel to pat dry the chicken and season the meat with paprika, salt and pepper.
5. Place a 12-inch cast-iron skillet over medium-high flame.
6. Add oil in the pan and make sure it completely covers the inside of the pan.
7. Place the chicken skin side down in the pan and cook for 8 minutes until golden.
8. Place the hot pan with the chicken in the oven and bake at 500 degrees F for 7 minutes.
9. Change sides and cook for 4 minutes until the chicken is tender and golden.

Nutrition (Per Serving): Calories: 332Fat: 22g Carbohydrates: 0g Protein: 31g Fiber: 0g Sugar: 0gSodium: 436mg

Tip: Serve the chicken thighs with salad for it to be extra filling, or a veggie side dish.

37. Bacon with Brussels Sprouts

Prep Time: 15 minutes
Cook Time: 15 minutes
Servings: 6

Ingredients:

- 1 ½ pounds Brussels sprouts, trimmed & halved
- 6 slices center-cut bacon, chopped
- 6 garlic cloves, thinly-sliced
- ½ cup sliced shallot
- ¾ cup fat-free & low-sodium chicken broth
- ⅛ teaspoon salt
- ⅛ teaspoon freshly ground black pepper

Instructions:
1. Place a large nonstick skillet over medium-high flame.
2. Cook and sauté bacon for 5 minutes or until browned.
3. Remove the pan from heat and take out the bacon from the skillet.
4. Use a slotted spot to reserve a tablespoon of drippings in pan while discarding the rest of the drippings.
5. Place the pan again on medium-high flame and sauté bacon, Brussels sprouts, and shallot for 4 minutes.
6. Stir in garlic and sauté for 4 minutes or until browned and fragrant.
7. Pour in the broth and let it come to a boil over high heat.
8. Cook until the broth mostly evaporated for about 2 minutes and the sprouts are crispy and tender—stir occasionally.
9. Remove pan from flame and stir in salt and pepper.
10. Serve out in a serving bowl and enjoy!

Nutrition (Per Serving): Calories: 90Fat: 2g Carbohydrates: 14g Protein: 7g Fiber: 0g Sugar: 0gSodium: 263mg

Tip: If you don't prefer throwing away the drippings, store them in a heatproof container and cool them before freezing them. You can utilize it as a replacement for cooking oil or fat.

38. Meatballs & Garlic-Lemon Orzo

Prep Time: 35 minutes

Cook Time: 10 minutes
Servings: 4

Ingredients:
- 1 pound ground lamb/beef
- 1 cup whole-wheat orzo
- 1 cup crumbled feta cheese, divided
- 1 cup cucumbers, thinly-sliced
- ½ cup whole-milk plain yogurt
- 1 large egg, lightly beaten
- 1 lemon zest & juice
- 4 tablespoons chopped fresh parsley, divided
- 3 tablespoons extra-virgin olive oil
- 2 tablespoons fresh dill, chopped
- 1 tablespoon fresh mint, chopped
- 3 teaspoons finely-grated garlic, divided
- ½ teaspoon salt

Instructions:
1. Start by preheating the oven at 425 degrees F.
2. Grease a large rimmed baking sheet with cooking spray.
3. Meanwhile, mix ground meat with egg, 2 tablespoons parsley, a teaspoon garlic and salt in a bowl.
4. Shape into 12 meatballs and arrange on the prepared baking sheet.
5. Bake for 20 minutes until cooked through and browned.
6. Meanwhile, take a large pan of water and let it come to a boil on high heat.
7. Cook orzo in it according to the package directions.
8. Drain and let it rest for 5 minutes.
9. Take a medium bowl and mix dill, remaining parsley, 2 teaspoons garlic, lemon zest, oil, and lemon juice.
10. Add a tablespoon of this mixture into a small bowl with yogurt and ¼ cup feta.
11. Transfer the orzo into the medium bowl and mix in the remaining ¾ cup feta.
12. Serve the meatballs with cucumbers, yogurt sauce and orzo.

Nutrition (Per Serving): Calories: 586Fat: 35g Carbohydrates: 37g Protein: 32g Fiber: 8g Sugar: 3gSodium: 649mg

Tip: You can add more salad veggies you like to this dish, for example cherry tomatoes and onions.

39. Sweet & Spicy Pork Kebabs

Prep Time: 25 minutes
Cook Time: 15 minutes
Servings: 4

Ingredients:
- 1 pound pork tenderloin, cut-into-1-inch-cubes
- 1 large red onion, cut-into-16-wedges
- 4 medium nectarines, quartered
- ¼ cup hoisin sauce
- 3 tablespoons mirin
- 1 tablespoon canola oil
- 1 tablespoon Chile-garlic sauce
- ½ teaspoon ground pepper
- ¼ teaspoon salt

Instructions:
1. Start by preheating the grill at medium-high.
2. Mix mirin, hoisin, and Chile-garlic sauce in a small bowl.
3. Save two tablespoons for serving later.
4. Take eight metal skewers of 12 inches and alternate between pork, onion, and nectarine pieces.
5. Brush with oil and season with salt and pepper.
6. Grill the kebabs from each side for 3 minutes or until browned.
7. Keep cooking and changing sides while brushing with the hoisin sauce.
8. Once the meat thermometer inserted into the thickest part of the meat reads 145• F, in about 10 minutes, it's done.
9. Brush the meat with the reserved hoisin sauce before serving.

Nutrition (Per Serving): Calories: 297 Fat: 7g Carbohydrates: 30g Protein: 26g Fiber: 4g Sugar: 21g Sodium: 537mg

Tip: If you want to bump up the tanginess of the meat, add lemon juice.

40. Grilled Steak with Salad Dressing

Prep Time: 10 minutes
Cook Time: 10 minutes
Servings: 4

Ingredients:
- 1 pound sirloin steak, trimmed
- 1 (11 oz.) package mixed greens
- 1 medium sweet onion, possibly Vidalia, cut-into-8-wedges
- 1 corn, husked
- 1 medium cucumber, sliced
- ¼ cup finely chopped fresh herbs, such as chives/dill/basil
- ¼ cup sunflower seeds
- 5 tablespoons extra-virgin olive oil, divided
- 2 tablespoons red wine vinegar
- 1 teaspoon Dijon mustard
- ¾ teaspoon salt, divided
- ½ teaspoon ground pepper, divided

Instructions:
1. Start by preheating the grill at medium-high.
2. Brush a tablespoon of oil on onion and corn.
3. Sprinkle ¼ teaspoon of salt and pepper on the steak.
4. Grease the grill rack with oil.
5. Grill the onion and corn, changing sides occasionally, for 8 minutes until they are tender and charred.
6. Next, grill the steak for 6-8 minutes until the thickest part reveals 125• on the medium-rare on an instant meat thermometer.
7. Remove the cooked steak on a cutting board and let cool for 5 minutes.
8. Cut the kernels from the corn.
9. Add vinegar, mustard, 2 onion wedges, ¼ teaspoon pepper, ½ teaspoon salt, and 4 tablespoons oil into a blender.
10. Blend until smooth and remove the dressing to a bowl.
11. Add corn, cucumber, mixed greens, remaining onion wedges, and herbs in the dressing bowl.
12. Toss to coat and slice the steak.
13. Serve the steak on top of the dressing mixture and garnish with sunflower seeds.

Nutrition (Per Serving): Calories: 409 Fat: 27g Carbohydrates: 17g Protein: 27g Fiber: 4g Sugar: 7g Sodium: 544mg

Tip: Use a grill basket to grill the onions. Otherwise, they can fall through the gaps between the grill grates.

Chapter 08: Fish & Seafood

41. Salmon Piccata with Sauce

Prep Time: 5 minutes
Cook Time: 10 minutes
Servings: 4

Ingredients:
- 1 ¼ pounds skin-on wild Alaskan salmon fillet, cut-into-4-portions
- ¼ cup dry white wine
- ¼ cup cold water
- 3 tablespoons shallot, minced
- 2 tablespoons extra-virgin olive oil, divided
- 2 tablespoons fresh lemon juice
- 2 tablespoons fresh parsley, finely-chopped
- 1 tablespoon capers, rinsed
- 1 tablespoon unsalted butter
- 1 teaspoon lemon zest, grated
- ½ teaspoon cornstarch
- ½ teaspoon kosher salt
- ⅛ teaspoon cracked black pepper

Instructions:
1. Place a large cast-iron skillet over medium-high flame with a tablespoon of oil for heating.
2. Use paper towels to pat dry salmon and season with salt and pepper.
3. Transfer salmon to the skillet, skin-side down, and lower heat to a medium to cook.
4. Use a spatula to press gently on the fish so its skin stays in contact with the hot pan firmly.
5. Give it 6-8 minutes to cook until it looks crispy and sides beginning to appear opaque.
6. Change sides and switch the heat to a low, and cook the salmon for a minute more until cooked through.
7. Remove to a plate and cover with foil.
8. Add the remaining tablespoon of oil to the pan with shallot.
9. Stir occasionally and cook until the shallot is fragrant and golden-brown.
10. Add in wine, stir and cook for a minute, until it's reduced to half.
11. Mix cornstarch and water in a small bowl and add to the pan.
12. Stir continuously until the sauce thickens in about a minute.
13. Take the pan off from heat and add in the capers, but smash them gently first with the back of a spoon.
14. Mix in lemon juice and zest, and swirl the butter in the pan until it is completely melted.
15. Serve the salmon with this sauce and parsley on top.

Nutrition (Per Serving): Calories: 312Fat: 19g Carbohydrates: 3g Protein: 29g Fiber: 1g Sugar: 1gSodium: 328mg

Tip: If dry white vinegar is unavailable, you can use white wine vinegar or chicken or vegetable broth instead.

42. Quick Crispy Salmon

Prep Time: 10 minutes
Cook Time: 15 minutes
Servings: 4

Ingredients:
- 4 (5 oz.) skin-on salmon fillets
- 2 tablespoons canola oil
- 1 tablespoon dry mustard
- 1 teaspoon garlic powder
- 1 teaspoon onion powder
- 1 teaspoon dried dill
- ½ teaspoon salt
- ¼ teaspoon celery seed
- Fresh dill fronds, for garnish

Instructions:
1. Place a large skillet over medium-high flame and heat oil.
2. Meanwhile, mix dill, garlic powder, dry mustard, onion powder, salt and celery seed in a small bowl.

3. Use paper towels to pat dry salmon and marinate it with the bowl mixture.
4. Place the salmon, skin-side down, onto the pan and cook for 3-4 minutes until crispy.
5. Flip and cook the other side for 4-6 minutes until cooked through and golden-brown.
6. Remove to a serving plate and garnish with fresh dill fronds if you like.

Nutrition (Per Serving): Calories: 277Fat: 17g Carbohydrates: 2g Protein: 29g Fiber: 0g Sugar: 0gSodium: 355mg

Tip: If you don't have dried mustard and dill, you can use regular mustard with herbs of your choice.

43. Simple Blackened Catfish

Prep Time: 10 minutes
Cook Time: 25 minutes
Servings: 4

Ingredients:
- 4 (5 oz.) skinless catfish fillets
- ½ cup salt-free blackening/Cajun seasoning
- ¼ cup loosely-packed fresh herb leaves, parsley/mint/chervil
- 1 tablespoon olive oil
- 1 tablespoon sweet/smoked sweet paprika
- 1 tablespoon freshly ground black pepper
- 2 tablespoons unsalted butter
- 1 teaspoon garlic powder/garlic salt
- 1 teaspoon onion powder
- 1 teaspoon ground dried oregano
- 1 teaspoon ground dried thyme or rosemary
- ¾ teaspoon kosher salt
- A pinch cayenne peppers
- Lemon wedges

Instructions:
1. Place a large cast-iron pan over high flame.
2. Meanwhile, mix black pepper, blackening seasoning, onion powder, paprika, oregano, thyme, cayenne, and garlic powder in a small bowl.
3. Season fish with salt and drizzle oil, and let it rest for 20 minutes.
4. Add ¼ blackening seasoning over the fish evenly, and press it into the fish.
5. Add butter to the hot pan and swirl it, so it covers the entire pan.
6. Cook the fish in the pan for 3-4 minutes.
7. Flip and cook the other side for another 2-3 minutes.
8. Once the fish is crusty, crispy, golden-brown and flaky, it's done.
9. Remove the fish to serving plates and season with fresh herbs evenly, and garnish with lemon wedges.

Nutrition (Per Serving): Calories: 251Fat: 18g Carbohydrates: 0g Protein: 22g Fiber: 0g Sugar: 0gSodium: 502mg

Tip: Also, you can heat a heavy cast-iron on the grill to cook the fish. Also, if you don't have fresh lemon juice available, you can use a bottled one instead.

44. Seasoned Grilled Red Snapper Fish

Prep Time: 10 minutes
Cook Time: 25 minutes
Servings: 4

Ingredients:
- 4 (5 oz.) boneless, skinless red snapper fillets
- 1 tablespoon extra-virgin olive oil
- 1 tablespoon smoked paprika
- 1 teaspoon onion powder
- 1 teaspoon garlic powder
- 1 teaspoon dried oregano
- 1 teaspoon dried thyme
- 1 teaspoon ground pepper
- ½ teaspoon salt
- ½ teaspoon cayenne pepper

- Lemon wedges, for garnish

Instructions:
1. Start by preheating the grill at medium-high typically between 400-450 degrees F.
2. Mix cayenne, thyme, oregano, onion powder, garlic powder, paprika, salt and pepper in a bowl.
3. Brush oil over the fish and season with the seasoning and press it into the skin.
4. Brush oil over the grill and cook the fish until it flakes effortlessly for 3-5 minutes each side.
5. Insert the meat thermometer in the thickest portion of the fish, if it reads 145 degrees F, it's done!
6. Remove to serving platter and garnish with lemon wedges.

Nutrition (Per Serving): Calories: 185Fat: 6g Carbohydrates: 3g Protein: 30g Fiber: 1g Sugar: 0gSodium: 384mg

Tip: You can grill your favorite veggies to, like onions, and broccoli, to have with the fish.

45. Crusted Sweet Scallops

Prep Time: 10 minutes
Cook Time: 25 minutes
Servings: 4

Ingredients:
- 1-pound large dry sea scallops
- 1 oz. Parmesan cheese, low-fat, grated
- ½ cup whole-wheat panko breadcrumbs
- 3 tablespoons olive oil, divided
- 2 tablespoons lemon juice
- 2 tablespoons shallot, chopped
- 2 tablespoons unsalted butter, melted
- 2 tablespoons chopped fresh flat-leaf parsley
- ¼ teaspoon kosher salt
- ¼ teaspoon ground pepper

Instructions:

1. Start by preheating the oven at 425 degrees F.
2. Take an 8-inch square baking pan and coat with a tablespoon of oil.
3. Use paper towels to pat scallops dry and place them in the baking dish in a single layer.
4. Season them with salt and pepper evenly.
5. Take a small bowl and mix butter, shallot, and lemon juice.
6. Pour the mixture over the scallops.
7. Add panko in the same mixture bowl with remaining oil, Parmesan and parsley.
8. Sprinkle this mixture over the scallops evenly.
9. Bake the scallops for 10-15 minutes until golden-brown and opaque.
10. Remove to serving plates and serve immediately.

Nutrition (Per Serving): Calories: 281Fat: 18g Carbohydrates: 13g Protein: 17g Fiber: 1g Sugar: 1gSodium: 407mg

Tip: If you don't have scallops, use onion powder instead. Or simply substitute with minced garlic.

46. Panko & Pistachio Crusted Halibut

Prep Time: 10 minutes
Cook Time: 10 minutes
Servings: 4

Ingredients:
- 1 ¼ pounds halibut, cut-into-4-portions
- 1 large garlic clove, grated
- 3 tablespoons unsalted pistachios, chopped
- 3 tablespoons panko breadcrumbs
- 1 tablespoon low-fat mayonnaise
- ½ teaspoon kosher salt
- ¼ teaspoon ground pepper

Instructions:
1. Start by preheating the oven at 425 degrees F.
2. Take a baking sheet and grease it with cooking spray.
3. Use paper towels to pat dry halibut fillets and arrange on the baking sheet.
4. Brush mayonnaise over the top of the fillets.
5. Meanwhile, mix panko, pistachios and garlic in a small bowl.
6. Spread this mixture over the fillets evenly and press the mixture to make it stick to the fish.
7. Bake for 10-12 minutes until the fillets flake easily with a fork.
8. Remove to serving plates and serve immediately.

Nutrition (Per Serving): Calories: 189Fat: 6g Carbohydrates: 5g Protein: 28g Fiber: 1g Sugar: 1gSodium: 367mg

Tip: If you don't prefer Halibut or its unavailable, you can use cod, tilapia, and haddock instead. Serve the fillets with lemon wedges for extra flavor!

47. One Pot Shrimp with Spinach

Prep Time: 10 minutes
Cook Time: 15 minutes
Servings: 4

Ingredients:
- 1 pound shrimp, peeled & deveined
- 1 pound spinach
- 6 medium sliced garlic cloves, divided
- 3 tablespoons extra-virgin olive oil, divided
- 1 tablespoon lemon juice
- 1 tablespoon fresh parsley, finely-chopped
- 1 ½ teaspoons lemon zest
- ¼ teaspoon crushed red pepper
- ¼ teaspoon salt + ⅛ teaspoon, divided

Instructions:
1. Place a large pot over medium flame and heat a tablespoon of oil.
2. Stir in half garlic and cook until browned for a minute or two.
3. Stir in spinach and ¼ salt and toss to combine.
4. Once spinach is mostly wilted, remove pan from heat and mix in lemon juice.
5. Remove to a bowl and let it keep warm.
6. Return the pot to the stove and increase the heat to medium-high.
7. Add two tablespoons of oil and stir in remaining garlic until browned.
8. Stir in remaining ⅛ teaspoon salt, shrimp, and crushed red pepper.
9. Stir and cook the shrimp for 3-5 minutes until cooked through.
10. Remove the shrimp to a serving plate and serve with spinach and topped with lemon zest and parsley.

Nutrition (Per Serving): Calories: 226Fat: 12g Carbohydrates: 6g Protein: 26g Fiber: 3g Sugar: 1gSodium: 444mg

48. One Pot Shrimp & Broccoli

Prep Time: 10 minutes
Cook Time: 10 minutes
Servings: 4

Ingredients:
- 1-pound raw shrimp, peeled & deveined
- 4 cups small broccoli florets
- 6 medium sliced garlic cloves
- 3 tablespoons extra-virgin olive oil, divided
- 2 teaspoons lemon juice, more as needed
- ½ teaspoon salt, divided
- ½ teaspoon ground pepper, divided

Instructions:
1. Place a large pot over medium flame and heat 2 tablespoons oil.
2. Stir in half garlic and cook for a minute until browned.
3. Stir in broccoli, ¼ teaspoon of salt and pepper.
4. Close the lid and cook for 3-5 minutes, and keep adding a tablespoon of water if the pan gets too dry, until the veggies become soft.
5. Remove to a bowl and let it keep warm.
6. Return pot to the stove and increase heat to medium-high.
7. Add the remaining tablespoon of oil and cook garlic for a minute until browned.
8. Add in shrimps with remaining ¼ teaspoon salt and pepper and cook for 3-5 minutes, while stirring, until tender.
9. Add the broccoli mixture into the shrimp with lemon juice and stir to combine.
10. Remove to serving bowls and serve immediately.

Nutrition (Per Serving): Calories: 214Fat: 11g Carbohydrates: 6g Protein: 25g Fiber: 2g Sugar: 2gSodium: 441mg

Tip: Serve this with rice, fried cauliflower rice, or noodles to make it more filling.

49. Mediterranean-Style Cod with Tomatoes

Prep Time: 10 minutes
Cook Time: 20 minutes
Servings: 4

Ingredients:
- 1 pound cod fillet
- 1 cup cherry tomatoes, halved
- ¼ cup cured olives, chopped
- 1 tablespoon shallot, minced
- 1 tablespoon capers, rinsed & chopped
- 3 teaspoons extra-virgin olive oil, divided
- 1 ½ teaspoons fresh oregano, chopped
- 1 teaspoon balsamic vinegar
- ¼ teaspoon freshly ground pepper

Instructions:
1. Start by preheating the oven at 450 degrees F.
2. Take a baking sheet and grease with a cooking spray.
3. Marinate cod with 2 tablespoons oil and season with pepper.
4. Arrange cod on the baking sheet and place in the oven.
5. Roast for 15-20 minutes until it flakes easily with a fork, according to its thickness.
6. Meanwhile, heat the remainder of a tablespoon of oil in a small skillet over medium flame.
7. Stir in shallots and cook for 30 seconds until soft.
8. Stir in tomatoes and cook for 2-3 minutes and mix in vinegar, capers, cured olives, vinegar and oregano.
9. Remove pan from heat and serve the cod with this sauce.

Nutrition (Per Serving): Calories: 151Fat: 8g Carbohydrates: 4g Protein: 16g Fiber: 1g Sugar: 1gSodium: 588mg

Tip: If you don't have shallots available, use regular onion and garlic instead

50. Crispy Pan-Fried White Bass

Prep Time: 10 minutes
Cook Time: 10 minutes
Servings: 4

Ingredients:
- 4 (6 oz.) bass fillets, skinned
- 1 large egg white
- ¼ cup seasoned breadcrumbs
- 2 tablespoons cornmeal
- 1 tablespoon all-purpose flour
- 1 tablespoon water
- 2 teaspoons vegetable oil
- 1 teaspoon butter
- ¼ teaspoon salt
- ¼ teaspoon black pepper
- 4 lemon wedges, for garnish

Instructions:
1. Place a large nonstick skillet over medium flame.
2. Mix flour, salt and pepper in a large plastic zip bag.
3. Take a shallow dish and mix egg white with water.
4. In another bowl, mix breadcrumbs and cornmeal with a whisk.
5. First, coat the fish with the zip bag mixture by shaking.
6. Next, dip it in egg white mixture and coat with the breadcrumb's mixture.
7. Repeat this process with the remaining fillets.
8. Add vegetable oil and butter to the pan and wait for the butter to melt.
9. Cook fillets in the pan for 5 minutes on each side until they flake easily with a fork.
10. Remove to a serving platter and serve with lemon wedges.

Nutrition (Per Serving): Calories: 250Fat: 8g Carbohydrates: 11g Protein: 33g Fiber: 0g Sugar: 0gSodium: 485mg

Tip: Serve this fish with your favorite steamed veggies or rice to make it more filling.

51. Hearty Shrimp & Fish Stew

Prep Time: 10 minutes
Cook Time: 20 minutes
Servings: 2

Ingredients:
- 8 oz. skinless cod or sea bass fillets
- 6 oz. raw shrimp, peeled & deveined
- 1 (14.5 oz.) can salt-free diced tomatoes, drained
- 1 (8 oz.) can salt-free tomato sauce
- 2 celery stalks, sliced
- 1 cup low-sodium chicken broth
- ¼ cup dry white wine/low-sodium chicken broth
- ⅓ cup onion, chopped
- 1 tablespoon snipped fresh parsley
- 2 teaspoons extra-virgin olive oil
- 1 teaspoon dried oregano, crushed
- ½ teaspoon garlic, minced
- ¼ teaspoon salt
- ⅛ teaspoon ground black pepper

Instructions:
1. Place a large saucepan over medium flame to heat oil.
2. But before that, cut the fish into 1 ½ inch pieces, and the shrimp in half lengthwise.
3. And refrigerate them for use later.
4. Cook onion, garlic, and celery in the hot oil pan for 5 minutes until tender.
5. Stir in a cup of broth and wine gently and let it come to a boil.
6. Mix in tomato sauce, drained tomatoes, oregano, salt and pepper.

7. Bring it to a boil once again and lower heat to a simmer.
8. Close the lid and let it cook for 5 minutes.
9. Carefully add fish and shrimp while stirring.
10. Return to a boil and lower the heat to a simmer quickly.
11. Close the lid and leave it to a simmer for 4-6 minutes until the fish flakes easily with a fork.
12. Remove this to serving plates and garnish with parsley on top.

Nutrition (Per Serving): Calories: 327Fat: 18g Carbohydrates: 22g Protein: 6g Fiber: 3g Sugar: 1gSodium: 759mg

Tip: If shrimps are not your cup of tea, you can add any white fish in this recipe.

52. Simple Baked Fish Fillets

Prep Time: 10 minutes
Cook Time: 20 minutes
Servings: 4

Ingredients:
- 1 ½ pounds cod
- ½ cup fresh breadcrumbs
- 2 tablespoons fresh parsley, chopped
- 1 ½ tablespoons butter/stick margarine, melted
- 1 tablespoon fresh lime juice
- 1 tablespoon light mayonnaise
- ⅛ teaspoon onion powder
- ⅛ teaspoon black pepper
- Cooking spray as needed

Instructions:
1. Start by preheating the oven at 425 degrees F.
2. Take a 11x7 inch baking dish and grease it with cooking spray, and place the fish inside.
3. Meanwhile, mix onion powder, lime juice, mayonnaise, and pepper and rub over the fish evenly.
4. Sprinkle breadcrumbs over the fish evenly and drizzle with butter.
5. Bake for 20 minutes until the fish is cooked through and flakes easily with a fork.
6. Remove from the pan and serve with parsley sprinkled on top.

Nutrition (Per Serving): Calories: 223Fat: 8g Carbohydrates: 5g Protein: 34g Fiber: 0g Sugar: 0gSodium: 223mg

Tip: To make the fish even more satisfying, bake potatoes with it or have with your favorite steamed greens.

53. Calamari with Fresh Herbs Salad

Prep Time: 20 minutes
Cook Time: 0 minutes
Servings: 4

Ingredients:
- 1-pound cleaned squid (tubes & tentacles), rinsed
- ½ cup red onion, thinly-sliced
- ½ cup roasted red peppers, thinly-sliced
- ½ cup cherry tomatoes, chopped
- ¼ cup celery, chopped
- ¼ cup extra-virgin olive oil
- 2 tablespoons fresh flat-leaf parsley, chopped
- 2 tablespoons fresh dill, chopped
- 2 tablespoons fresh lemon juice
- 2 tablespoons white wine vinegar
- 1 tablespoon Kalamata olives, finely-chopped & pitted
- ¼ teaspoon salt
- ¼ teaspoon ground pepper

Instructions:
1. Place a large pot of water on high heat and bring to a boil.
2. Prepare a bowl of ice water and set near the stove.
3. Slice squid tubes into ¼ inch thick slices and keep the tentacles whole.
4. Put the chopped squid tubes and whole tentacles into the boiling water.
5. Cook for a minute without stirring.
6. Then with a large slotted spoon, remove them to the bowl of ice water.
7. Let it cool for 5 minutes until opaque and drain well afterwards.
8. Meanwhile, mix vinegar, lemon juice, oil, parsley, dill, olives, salt and pepper in a bowl.
9. Lastly, add onion, cooled calamari, tomatoes, celery, and roasted red peppers.
10. Toss everything to combine and serve once the flavors have melded well.

Nutrition (Per Serving): Calories: 269Fat: 18g Carbohydrates: 9g Protein: 18g Fiber: 1g Sugar: 3gSodium: 463mg

Tip: You can refrigerate this salad for up to 2 days.

54. Fish Fillets with Lemon-Dill Sauce

Prep Time: 15 minutes
Cook Time: 15 minutes
Servings: 4

Ingredients:
- 4 (6 oz.) skinless cod fillets
- 2 large egg whites, lightly-beaten
- 1 cup panko breadcrumbs
- ¼ cup canola mayonnaise
- 2 tablespoons dill pickle, finely-chopped
- 1 teaspoon fresh lemon juice
- 1 teaspoon fresh dill, chopped
- 1 teaspoon black pepper
- ½ teaspoon paprika
- ¾ teaspoon onion powder
- ¾ teaspoon garlic powder
- ⅜ teaspoon salt
- Cooking spray, as needed
- Lemon wedges, as garnish

Instructions:
1. Start by preheating the broiler to high heat.
2. Add egg whites in a shallow dish.
3. Meanwhile, mix paprika, panko, garlic powder, and onion powder.
4. Season the fish fillets with salt and pepper evenly.
5. Then dunk each fish fillet in egg white and coat with the panko mixture and place them on the broiler pan greased with cooking spray.
6. Broil the fish fillets each side for 4 minutes until cooked through and crispy.
7. Meanwhile, mix dill, mayonnaise, lemon juice, and pickle in a small bowl.

8. Garnish the fish with lemon wedges and serve with the mayonnaise sauce!

Nutrition (Per Serving): Calories: 245Fat: 5g Carbohydrates: 12g Protein: 35g Fiber: 0g Sugar: 0gSodium: 580mg

Tip: You can substitute Cod with Halibut or Tilapia in case of unavailability.

55. Salmon & Peppercorn Sauce

Prep Time: 10 minutes
Cook Time: 15 minutes
Servings: 4

Ingredients:
- 1 ¼ pounds wild salmon fillet, skinned & cut-into-4-portions
- ¼ cup lemon juice
- 4 teaspoons unsalted butter, cubed
- 2 teaspoons canola oil
- 1 teaspoon green peppercorns in vinegar, rinsed & crushed
- ¼ teaspoon + a pinch salt, divided

Instructions:
1. Place a large nonstick skillet over medium-high flame and heat oil.
2. Season salmon fillets with ¼ teaspoon salt.
3. Cook salmon fillets for 4-7 minutes both sides until opaque in the middle.
4. Remove to serving plates and take the pan off from heat.
5. Add peppercorn, butter, lemon juice, and the remaining pinch of salt to the pan and swirl the pan till coated from all sides.
6. Spoon sauce over the salmon carefully and serve immediately.

Nutrition (Per Serving): Calories: 226Fat: 11g Carbohydrates: 1g Protein: 28g Fiber: 0g Sugar: 0gSodium: 269mg

Tip: If green peppercorns aren't available, fresh ground black pepper works fine as well.

Chapter 09: Vegetarian & Vegan Dishes

56. Toasted Shishito Peppers

Prep Time: 5 minutes
Cook Time: 10 minutes
Servings: 4

Ingredients:
- 12 oz. fresh shishito peppers
- ¼ cup low-fat mayonnaise
- 1 large garlic clove, grated
- 1 ½ tablespoons toasted sesame oil, divided
- 1 tablespoon lime juice, divided
- 1 teaspoon toasted sesame seeds
- ¼ teaspoon flaky sea salt
- Lime wedges, for garnish

Instructions:
1. Place a large cast-iron skillet over medium-high flame.
2. Mix garlic, mayonnaise and 1 ½ teaspoon of lime juice and sesame oil in a small bowl.
3. Layer the peppers in the hot pan and cook for 3 minutes until it begins to char
4. Continue cooking for 4-6 minutes more until peppers are charred from each side.
5. Meanwhile, mix the remaining ½ teaspoon lime juice and 1 tablespoon sesame oil in a large bowl.
6. Add in the hot peppers and a sprinkle of sesame seeds and flaky sea salt on top.
7. Toss to combine and transfer to a serving plate.
8. Garnish with lime wedges and serve with the mayo-garlic sauce.

Nutrition (Per Serving): Calories: 111Fat: 9g Carbohydrates: 7g Protein: 1g Fiber: 2g Sugar: 3gSodium: 273mg

Tip: Have these toasted peppers as a side dish or as a quick and healthy appetizer.

57. Burrata Pasta with Cherry Tomatoes

Prep Time: 10 minutes
Cook Time: 20 minutes
Servings: 4

Ingredients:
- 8 oz. whole-wheat fettuccine *or* linguine
- 8 oz. burrata cheese, low-fat
- 3 cups cherry tomatoes, halved
- 3 cups packed baby spinach
- ¼ cup extra-virgin olive oil
- ¼ cup chopped fresh basil, plus more for garnish
- 1 ½ tablespoons garlic, finely-chopped
- ½ teaspoon salt-free Italian seasoning
- ½ teaspoon crushed red pepper
- ¼ teaspoon salt
- ¼ teaspoon ground pepper

Instructions:
1. Place a large saucepan filled with water over high flame.
2. Bring it a boil and cook the pasta following the package directions.
3. Save ½ cup pasta water, drain well and put aside.
4. Next, heat oil over medium flame in a large high-sided skillet.
5. Stir in crushed red pepper, Italian seasoning, and garlic and cook for a minute or two until fragrant.
6. Add in tomatoes, stir and cook for 8-10 minutes until the tomatoes break down and become saucy.
7. Stir in salt and pepper and remove the pan from heat.
8. Add pasta and the saved water to the tomato skillet and toss to coat.
9. Stir in spinach and basil and toss to combine.

10. Return the skillet to medium flame and let it cook for 2 minutes until the pasta is properly mixed and the spinach has wilted.
11. Cut or tear the burrata into pieces and stir in the pasta.
12. Divide the pasta among serving plates and garnish with more basil to serve.

Nutrition (Per Serving): Calories: 498Fat: 30g Carbohydrates: 49g Protein: 20g Fiber: 7g Sugar: 5gSodium: 344mg

58. Moo-Shu Chinese Style Vegetables

Prep Time: 10 minutes
Cook Time: 10 minutes
Servings: 4

Ingredients:
- 1 (12 oz.) packed bag shredded mixed vegetables, like rainbow salad/broccoli slaw
- 1 bunch sliced scallions, divided
- 4 whisked large eggs
- 2 garlic cloves, minced
- 2 cups mung bean sprouts
- 2 tablespoons hoisin sauce
- 1 tablespoon rice vinegar
- 1 tablespoon low-sodium soy sauce
- 3 teaspoons toasted sesame oil, divided
- 2 teaspoons fresh ginger, minced

Instructions:
1. Place a large nonstick skillet over medium flame and heat a tablespoon of oil.
2. Add in lightly-beaten eggs, stir and cook for 2-3 minutes until set and transfer to a plate.
3. Wipe the pan and return it to the stove over medium flame.
4. Heat the remaining oil and stir in ginger and garlic.
5. Cook for a minute until softened and fragrant, then add in shredded vegetables.
6. Also, add bean sprouts, ½ sliced scallions, soy sauce and vinegar and stir to mix well.
7. Close the lid and let it cook for 3 minutes until the vegetables become tender, stirring once or twice.
8. Add in the reserved eggs and hoisin sauce, stir and cook for 2-3 minutes uncovered.
9. Use the spoon to break apart the egg scramble and let it all get heated through.
10. Stir in the rest of the scallions and remove the pan from heat.
11. Transfer the mixture to a serving bowl and serve immediately.

Nutrition (Per Serving): Calories: 172Fat: 9g Carbohydrates: 15g Protein: 11g Fiber: 4g Sugar: 7gSodium: 366mg

Tip: You can use fresh vegetables than packed ones if you want to cook from scratch. This mix is also great for a tortilla wrap if you want this to be even more filling.

59. Garlic Pea Shoots Stir Fry

Prep Time: 10 minutes
Cook Time: 10 minutes
Servings: 6

Ingredients:
- 1 pound pea shoots/sprouts or broccoli or spinach shoots
- ¼ cup Shaoxing rice wine
- 3 tablespoons garlic, minced
- 2 tablespoons canola oil
- 2 tablespoons sesame oil
- ¾ teaspoon salt
- ¼ teaspoon ground white pepper

Instructions:
1. Place a large wok or flat-bottomed pan over medium flame and heat both canola and sesame oil.
2. Stir in garlic and sauté for a minute until soft and fragrant.
3. Add in pea shoots, rice wine, salt and white pepper.
4. Stir and cook for 3 minutes until the pea shoots become tender and wilted.
5. Serve immediately as a side dish or a quick healthy snack!

Nutrition (Per Serving): Calories: 150Fat: 10g Carbohydrates: 7g Protein: 2g Fiber: 2g Sugar: 3gSodium: 291mg

Tip: For those who don't know, Shaoxing is an Asian rice wine for use in cooking. If it's not available, substitute it with dry Sherry instead.

60. Spicy Broccoli Stir Fry

Prep Time: 15 minutes
Cook Time: 20 minutes
Servings: 4

Ingredients:
- 5 cups bite-sized broccoli florets
- ⅓ cup water
- ½ cup salt-free roasted peanuts
- 5 small dried red chile peppers (or red peppers)
- 2 scallions, sliced
- 2 tablespoons peanut oil
- 1 ½ tablespoons Chinese black vinegar (or balsamic vinegar)
- 1 tablespoon hoisin sauce
- 1 tablespoon garlic, minced
- 1 tablespoon fresh ginger, minced
- 2 teaspoons low-sodium soy sauce
- 2 teaspoons toasted sesame oil
- 2 teaspoons cornstarch
- ½ teaspoon Chinese five-spice powder

Instructions:
1. Place a large wok or nonstick skillet over medium-high flame and heat peanut oil.
2. Mix water, hoisin, vinegar, sesame oil, soy sauce, cornstarch, and five-spice powder in a small bowl thorough and put aside.
3. Stir broccoli in the hot pan and cook for 6 minutes until crispy tender.
4. Stir in ginger, garlic, scallions, and chiles and cook for half a second until fragrant.
5. Lower heat and pour in the sauce mixture.
6. Continue stirring until the mixture has thickened a bit and then remove the pan from heat.
7. Stir in peanuts and serve immediately as a side dish or a quick healthy snack!

Nutrition (Per Serving): Calories: 259Fat: 19g Carbohydrates: 18g Protein: 9g Fiber: 5g Sugar: 6gSodium: 212mg

61. Peanut Butter Broccoli Stir Fry

Prep Time: 5 minutes
Cook Time: 10 minutes
Servings: 6

Ingredients:
- 8 cups broccoli florets, 2-inch-pieces
- ½ cup yellow onion, sliced
- 3 medium cloves garlic, chopped
- 3 tablespoons smooth & natural peanut butter
- 2 ½ tablespoons low-sodium tamari
- 2 tablespoons toasted sesame oil
- 2 tablespoons rice vinegar
- 1 tablespoon light brown sugar
- 1 tablespoon toasted sesame seeds
- 1 teaspoon cornstarch

Instructions:
1. Bring a large pot with a steamer basket filled with 1 inch water to a boil.
2. Stir in broccoli, close the lid, and cook for 3-4 minutes until tender.
3. Meanwhile, place a large skillet over medium-high flame and heat oil.
4. Stir in onion, garlic, to cook for 3 minutes until softened.
5. Stir in the steamed broccoli and cook for 3 minutes while stirring.
6. Mix tamari, vinegar, peanut butter, sugar, and cornstarch in a small bowl until smooth.
7. Add to the vegetables and cook for a minute until the sauce thickens.
8. Sprinkle toasted sesame seeds on top and serve immediately!

Nutrition (Per Serving): Calories: 154Fat: 10g Carbohydrates: 12g Protein: 6g Fiber: 3g Sugar: 5gSodium: 346mg

Tip: This is a great recipe to sneak in more veggies into your diet or manage food leftovers before they go to waste.

62. Lemon Asparagus Stir Fry

Prep Time: 10 minutes
Cook Time: 15 minutes
Servings: 2

Ingredients:
- 1-pound asparagus, cut into pieces
- 1 garlic clove, finely-chopped
- 1 lemon zest & juice
- 2 tablespoons extra-virgin olive oil, divided
- ¼ teaspoon salt
- Ground pepper, as per taste

Instructions:
1. Bring a large pot with a steamer basket filled with an inch of water to a boil.
2. Add asparagus to a large bowl of water and swirl to get rid of any debris.
3. Transfer to a steamer basket and let them steam for 10 minutes.
4. Remove to a clean kitchen towel and pat dry.
5. Place a large skillet over medium heat and heat a tablespoon of oil.
6. Stir in the asparagus and cook for 2-3 minutes until it starts to brown.
7. Add the remaining oil with lemon zest, lemon juice, garlic, salt and pepper as per taste.
8. Stir and cook for 30 seconds until fragrant.
9. Serve immediately as a side dish or a quick healthy snack.

Nutrition (Per Serving): Calories: 112Fat: 7g Carbohydrates: 12g Protein: 2.7g Fiber: 5g Sugar: 1gSodium: 416mg

Tip: Have them with brown rice or quinoa if you want to make it even more filling.

63. Toasted Zucchini Stir Fry

Prep Time: 5 minutes
Cook Time: 5 minutes
Servings: 4

Ingredients:
- 3 medium zucchini, cut-into-2-¾-wedges
- 3 scallions, 1-inch-green-parts-only
- 2 tablespoons water
- 1 ½ tablespoons low-sodium soy sauce
- 1 tablespoon toasted sesame oil
- 1 tablespoon fresh ginger, grated
- 1 tablespoon Sriracha
- 1 tablespoon honey
- 1 ½ teaspoons cornstarch

Instructions:
1. Place a large nonstick skillet over medium-high flame and heat oil for 1-2 minutes.
2. Meanwhile, mix ginger with Sriracha, soy sauce, honey and cornstarch in a small bowl until smooth.
3. Add in zucchini in a single layer and cook, without stirring, for 2 minutes until lightly-browned.
4. Pour water, cook with the lid closed, for 2 minutes until zucchini is tender and looks bright green.
5. Lower heat to medium and stir in the ginger mixture to cook until it thickens.
6. Remove from pan to a plate, drizzle sesame oil, and sprinkle scallions on top.
7. Toss to combine and serve immediately.

Nutrition (Per Serving): Calories: 91Fat: 4g Carbohydrates: 13g Protein: 3g Fiber: 2g Sugar: 9gSodium: 335mg

Tip: Have this stir fry with noodles for a more fulfilling experience or on its own as a quick healthy snack.

64. Broccoli with Tofu Stir Fry

Prep Time: 10 minutes
Cook Time: 20 minutes
Servings: 4

Ingredients:
- 1 (14 oz.) package extra-firm water-packed tofu, drained
- 6 cups broccoli florets
- ½ cup vegetable broth/low-sodium chicken broth
- ¼ cup dry sherry/rice wine
- 3 tablespoons water
- 3 tablespoons cornstarch, divided
- 3 tablespoons low-sodium soy sauce
- 2 tablespoons canola oil, divided
- 2 tablespoons + 1 teaspoon sugar
- 1 tablespoon garlic, minced
- 1 tablespoon fresh ginger, minced
- ¼ teaspoon crushed red pepper, plus more as needed
- ¼ teaspoon salt

Instructions:
1. Place a large wok or non-stick skillet over medium-high flame and heat a tablespoon of oil.
2. Meanwhile, cut tofu into ¾ inch cubes and pat dry with a cloth, and season with salt.
3. Mix sherry or rice wine, broth, soy sauce, sugar, a tablespoon cornstarch, and crushed red pepper in a bowl and put aside.
4. Cook tofu cubes in the hot skillet for 3 minutes without stirring.
5. Then turn the side and cook for another 2-3 minutes until browned, while stirring.
6. Remove to a plate and lower the heat of the stove.
7. Add the remaining tablespoon of oil in the skillet with ginger and garlic.
8. Cook for 30 seconds until fragrant and add broccoli and water.
9. Close the lid and cook for 2-4 minutes until broccoli is crispy-tender.

10. Mix the reserved broth mixture and add to the pan.
11. Cook to thicken the sauce for 1-2 minutes.
12. Then add tofu to the pan mixture and toss to combine it all together.
13. Serve immediately and have with noodles if you like.

Nutrition (Per Serving): Calories: 257Fat: 13g Carbohydrates: 23g Protein: 14g Fiber: 4g Sugar: 7gSodium: 665mg

Tip: People careful about their gluten intake should only use soy sauces sold as gluten-free. Regular soy sauce may contain gluten-containing sweeteners and additions.

65. Chicken-Style Seitan Stir Fry

Prep Time: 10 minutes
Cook Time: 20 minutes
Servings: 2

Ingredients:
- 8 oz. water-packed Seitan, possibly chicken-style, drained & patted dry
- 2 carrots, peeled & thinly-sliced
- ¼ cup sherry
- ¼ cup water
- 2 tablespoons peanuts, chopped
- 2 tablespoons chopped fresh cilantro, optional
- 1 tablespoon hoisin sauce
- 1 tablespoon brown sugar
- 1 tablespoon lime juice
- 4 teaspoons canola oil, divided
- 1 teaspoon cornstarch
- 1 teaspoon fresh ginger, chopped
- ⅛ teaspoon salt

Instructions:
1. Place a large nonstick skillet over medium-high flame and heat 3 teaspoons of peanut oil.
2. Meanwhile, mix hoisin, sherry, water, cornstarch, brown sugar, lime and salt in a small bowl thoroughly.
3. Stir Seitan in the hot pan and cook for 4-7 minutes until crispy.
4. Add the remaining teaspoon of oil with peanuts and ginger, stir and cook for a minute until fragrant.
5. Stir in carrots and red pepper and cook for minutes while stirring.
6. Whisk the sauce in the small bowl and pour in the pan.
7. Stir to coat, cover the lid and let everything cook for 3 minutes until the vegetables are tender and sauce has melded well.
8. Garnish with cilantro if you like and serve immediately.

Nutrition (Per Serving): Calories: 353Fat: 15g Carbohydrates: 33g Protein: 20g Fiber: 12g Sugar: 14gSodium: 704mg

Tip: For those who don't know, Seitan is a meaty-textured product made from wheat gluten with a high protein content. It's usually found next to Tofu in health stores or big supermarkets. While buying, look for the "drained weight" as the package weight depends on whether the "water weight" has been considered.

66. Chinese green beans stir fry

Prep Time: 10 minutes
Cook Time: 10 minutes
Servings: 6

Ingredients:
- 4 (1 ½ pounds) green beans
- 2 jalapeño peppers, cut-into-thin-rings
- 1 small yellow onion, ¼-inch-wedge-cut-slices
- 1 cup packed fresh basil leaves
- 5 tablespoons canola oil/peanut oil, divided
- 2 tablespoons hoisin sauce
- 2 tablespoons low-sodium soy sauce
- 1 tablespoon plum sauce
- 2 teaspoons garlic, minced
- 1 teaspoon fresh ginger, minced

Instructions:
1. Place a large cast-iron skillet over high flame and heat 2 tablespoons oil.
2. Meanwhile, cut the green beans into quarters lengthwise, then into 2-inch pieces.
3. Add half of the pieces to the hot skillet and cook for 4-5 minutes until browned and tender, stirring frequently.
4. Remove to a large bowl and repeat the same process with the remaining green bean pieces.
5. Keep the green bean pieces warm by covering.
6. Meanwhile, mix soy sauce, hoisin, and plum sauce in a small bowl.
7. Heat a tablespoon of oil in the skillet over high flame.
8. Stir in jalapenos and onion, cook and sauté for 4-5 minutes until softened a bit and fragrant.
9. Then stir in ginger and garlic and cook for a minute.
10. Add this sauté to the reserved green beans with the sauce.
11. Stir to combine and serve immediately!

Nutrition (Per Serving): Calories: 161Fat: 12g Carbohydrates: 13g Protein: 2g Fiber: 2g Sugar: 6gSodium: 298mg

Tip: Keep the leftover stored in your refrigerator and reheat for 5 minutes before serving.

67. Creamy Brussels Sprouts with Fettuccine

Prep Time: 10 minutes
Cook Time: 20 minutes
Servings: 6

Ingredients:
- 12 oz. whole-wheat fettuccine
- 4 cups sliced mixed mushrooms, like cremini/oyster/shiitake
- 4 cups Brussels sprouts, thinly-sliced
- 2 cups low-fat milk
- 1 cup finely-shredded Asiago cheese, extra for garnish
- ½ cup dry sherry
- 2 tablespoons all-purpose flour
- 1 tablespoon extra-virgin olive oil
- 1 tablespoon garlic, minced
- ½ teaspoon salt
- ½ teaspoon freshly-ground pepper

Instructions:
1. Place a large pot of water over high heat and bring it to a boil.
2. Cook pasta for 8-10 minutes as per the package directions.
3. Drain well, return to the pot, and set aside for use later.
4. Meanwhile, place a large skillet over medium flame and heat oil.
5. Stir in mushrooms and Brussels sprouts to cook for 8-10 minutes until the mushrooms get mushy.
6. Stir in garlic for a minute and add sherry or vinegar.

7. Scrape any brown bits in there and let it reach a boil.
8. Then, cook for 10 seconds if using sherry or for a whole minute if using vinegar.
9. Meanwhile, mix flour and milk in a bowl and add to the skillet with salt and pepper.
10. Cook for 2 minutes while stirring until the sauce starts bubbling and to thicken.
11. Then mix in Asiago until it melts and add this mixture to the pasta.
12. Toss to combine and serve immediately with extra cheese, if you like.

Nutrition (Per Serving): Calories: 384Fat: 10g Carbohydrates: 56g Protein: 18g Fiber: 10g Sugar: 8gSodium: 431mg

Tip: Cooking Sherry contains a lot of sodium, so go with dry Sherry instead which doesn't have a high-sodium content.

68. Goat Cheese & Beet Pasta

Prep Time: 10 minutes
Cook Time: 15 minutes
Servings: 4

Ingredients:
- 12 oz. whole-wheat fettuccine/pappardelle
- 1 (6.5 oz.) package garlic-herb marinated baby beets, like Love Beets
- 4 oz. creamy goat cheese, divided
- ¼ cup toasted walnuts, coarsely-chopped
- ¼ cup fresh basil, chopped
- 6 tablespoons water
- 2 tablespoons extra-virgin olive oil
- 1 tablespoon white miso
- 1 tablespoon lemon zest
- ¼ teaspoon salt
- ¼ teaspoon ground pepper

Instructions:
1. Place a large pot of water over high flame and bring to a boil.
2. Cook fettuccine or pappardelle as per the package instructions.
3. Save ½ cup pasta water, drain well and set pasta and reserved water aside.
4. Meanwhile, add beets with oil, water, lemon zest, 2 oz. Goat cheese, white miso, salt and pepper in a blender.
5. Blend for a minute until smooth.
6. Crumble the rest of the 2oz. Goat cheese and put aside.
7. Transfer the blended sauce to a large skillet over medium flame and let it come to a simmer.
8. Toss in the pasta carefully while slowly adding the reserved pasta water, a tablespoon at a time to reach the desired consistency.
9. Toss to combine and divide the pasta among serving bowls.
10. Garnish with walnuts, basil and crumbled goat cheese and serve immediately.

Nutrition (Per Serving): Calories: 474Fat: 20g Carbohydrates: 51g Protein: 19g Fiber: 11g Sugar: 5gSodium: 427mg

Tip: If marinated baby beets are not available, regular ones will do. Also, add two teaspoons lemon juice to the pasta sauce to make up for the non-marinated beets.

69. Chickpea Salad with Cranberry & Walnut

Prep Time: 6 minutes
Cook Time: 4 minutes
Servings: 2

Ingredients:
- 1 (15 oz.) can salt-free chickpeas, rinsed
- ¼ cup low-fat plain & strained yogurt, like Greek-style
- ¼ cup celery, diced
- ¼ cup dried cranberries
- ¼ cup toasted walnuts, chopped
- 1 tablespoon onion, minced
- 2 teaspoons lemon juice
- ¼ teaspoon salt

Instructions:
1. Place a small dry skillet over medium-low flame.
2. Add in chopped walnuts and toast them for 2-4 minutes while stirring constantly.
3. Once they are golden-brown and fragrant, add it to the salad.
4. To make the salad, combine yogurt, lemon juice, onion and salt in a medium bowl.
5. Add celery, chickpeas, cranberries and toasted walnuts.
6. Toss it all to combine and serve immediately.

Nutrition (Per Serving): Calories: 396Fat: 12g Carbohydrates: 55g Protein: 17g Fiber: 11g Sugar: 18gSodium: 361mg

Tip: If you are allergic to walnuts, you can add your own choice of nuts.

70. Pineapple & Tofu Stir Fry

Prep Time: 10 minutes
Cook Time: 25 minutes
Servings: 2

Ingredients:
- 1 (8 oz.) can pineapple chunks/bits, save 3 tablespoons juice
- 7 oz. extra-firm, water-packed tofu, drained, rinsed, & cubed-into-½-pieces
- 1 tablespoon garlic, minced
- 1 tablespoon low-sodium soy sauce
- 1 tablespoon ketchup
- 5 teaspoons rice vinegar
- 3 teaspoons canola oil, divided
- 2 teaspoons brown sugar
- 2 teaspoons ginger, minced
- 1 teaspoon cornstarch

Instructions:
1. Place a large nonstick skillet over medium-high flame and heat 2 tablespoons of oil.
2. Meanwhile, mix the saved pineapple juice, soy sauce, vinegar, ketchup and sugar in a small bowl until smooth.
3. Add tofu in a separate medium bowl and combine with 2 tablespoons of the pineapple sauce.
4. Let it rest in the marination for 5 minutes.
5. Add cornstarch to the remaining pineapple sauce and mix thoroughly until smooth.
6. Add the tofu in the hot pan with a slotted spoon and add the remaining marinade in the pineapple sauce.
7. Cook the tofu for 7-9 minutes until golden-brown while stirring every 2 minutes.
8. Remove the tofu to a plate and set aside.
9. Heat the remaining oil in the skillet over medium flame.
10. Stir in garlic and ginger and cook for 30 seconds until fragrant.
11. Pour in the sauce, stir and cook until it starts to thicken for half a second.

12. Then add the tofu and pineapple sauce and cook for 2 additional minutes while stirring gently.
13. Serve immediately and enjoy!

Nutrition (Per Serving): Calories: 269Fat: 12g Carbohydrates: 35g Protein: 10g Fiber: 4g Sugar: 26gSodium: 363mg

Tip: Leftover tofu should be rinsed, put in a storage container with water and stored in the fridge. It'll last you 2-4 days if you change the water every day. Freezing tofu can also give you 5 months and more time to use, but it develops a chewy texture and a caramel shade in the process which is likened to personal preference

Grab Your Exclusive Bonuses in the Conclusion Chapter!

BONUS 1 - 30 Days Meal Plan Grocery List: Kickstart your health journey with a ready-made grocery list tailored for our meal plan. No guesswork, just grab and go!

BONUS 2 - Foods to Eat & Avoid Cards: A quick cheat sheet to keep your meals anti-inflammatory friendly. Know what to embrace and what to avoid at a glance.

BONUS 3 - Grocery List: A template featuring the most common healthy foods. Quickly jot down what you need for your recipes and take it shopping—effortless and efficient.

BONUS 4 - Recipe Card: Discover a new favorite? Note it down and make it a heart-healthy classic in your kitchen.

BONUS 5 - Weekly Meal Plan Template: Flex your culinary creativity with a customizable template.

The bonuses are 100% FREE – Check out the conclusion chapter to easily claim them

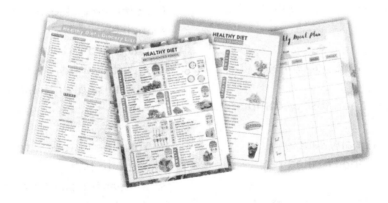

Your review can guide and inspire! If you've yet to share your thoughts on our cookbook, please consider doing so now. A photo with your review would beautifully highlight our collective journey towards heart health.

Help light the way to healthier living!!

Chapter 10: Snack Recipes

71. English Muffin with Tuna Salad

Prep Time: 10 minutes
Cook Time: 0 minutes
Servings: 1

Ingredients:

- 2 ½ oz. salt-free water-packed canned tuna, drained
- 1 toasted whole-wheat English muffin
- ¼ cup English cucumber, thinly-sliced
- 1 tablespoon mayonnaise
- 1 tablespoon scallion, thinly-sliced
- 1 teaspoon rice vinegar
- ¼ teaspoon honey
- ½ teaspoon low-sodium soy sauce
- ½ teaspoon Sriracha/other hot sauce
- ½ teaspoon toasted sesame oil
- A pinch crushed red pepper, optional

Instructions:
1. Combine soy sauce, honey, and vinegar together in a small bowl.
2. Add in cucumber slices and toss to combine and put aside.
3. Mix scallion, Sriracha or any sauce, mayonnaise, sesame oil, and crushed red pepper if desired.
4. Also stir in tuna and drain the cucumbers.
5. Spoon the tuna mixture over one muffin half and layer cucumbers on top.
6. Then cover the top with the other muffin top.
7. Plate it out and serve immediately!

Nutrition (Per Serving): Calories: 349Fat: 15g Carbohydrates: 31g Protein: 24g Fiber: 5g Sugar: 8gSodium: 572mg

Tip: Make sure to toast your English muffin, otherwise the sandwich will end up being soggy.

72. Crispy Green Lettuce Wraps with Turkey

Prep Time: 15 minutes
Cook Time: 0 minutes
Servings: 4

Ingredients:

- 12 oz. deli turkey, sliced
- 4 oz. deli sharp Cheddar cheese, low-fat, sliced
- 8 large green-leaf lettuce leaves
- 8 tomato slices
- ¼ cup mayonnaise
- 3 tablespoons dill pickle, chopped
- 2 teaspoons whole-grain mustard

Instructions:
1. Combine pickle, mustard, and mayonnaise in a small bowl.
2. Place two lettuce leaves on top of each other like a cross and spread a tablespoon of mayonnaise over the lettuce.
3. Add in 3 oz turkey, 1 oz cheese, and 2 tomato slices.
4. Turn the lettuce into a wrap by rolling and slice it into half.
5. Repeat the same process with the remaining lettuce leaves.
6. Serve immediately and enjoy your lunch!

Nutrition (Per Serving): Calories: 324Fat: 22g Carbohydrates: 3g Protein: 21g Fiber: 1g Sugar: 1gSodium: 827mg

Tip: These wraps are perfect when you are in a hurry and in need of a quick, healthy snack. You can use any other meat slices if you don't prefer turkey.

73. Healthy & Creamy Pesto Chicken

Prep Time: 15 minutes
Cook Time: 15 minutes
Servings: 4

Ingredients:
- 1 pound boneless & skinless chicken breast, trimmed
- 1 (5 oz.) package mixed salad greens
- 1 pint grape/cherry tomatoes, halved
- ¼ cup pesto
- ¼ cup low-fat mayonnaise
- 3 tablespoons red onion, finely-chopped
- 2 tablespoons extra-virgin olive oil
- 2 tablespoons red-wine vinegar
- ¼ teaspoon salt
- ¼ teaspoon ground pepper

Instructions:
1. Place a medium saucepan over medium flame.
2. Add chicken and 1 inch water to cover it.
3. Let it come to a boil and lower the heat to a gentle simmer for 10-15 minutes until chicken loses its raw, pink color.
4. Remove the chicken to a cutting board and shred into thin pieces once cool.
5. Meanwhile, mix mayonnaise, pesto, and onion in a medium bowl.
6. Mix in the shredded chicken and toss to coat.
7. Mix vinegar, oil, salt and pepper in a separate large bowl.
8. Add in the greens with tomatoes and toss to combine.
9. Serve the greens and tomatoes among 4 plates and place the chicken salad on top.

Nutrition (Per Serving): Calories: 324Fat: 20g Carbohydrates: 9g Protein: 27g Fiber: 2g Sugar: 3gSodium: 454mg

Tip: Instead of boiling, you can roast and bake the chicken to turn into shreds. This recipe also brings up the perfect opportunity to use your veggie leftovers to make this even more filling.

74. Black Beans & Veggie Taco Bowl

Prep Time: 10 minutes
Cook Time: 10 minutes
Servings: 1

Ingredients:
- 1 oz. sharp Cheddar cheese, low-fat, shredded
- ½ red onion, sliced
- ½ cup brown rice, cooked
- ¼ cup canned black beans, rinsed
- ¼ cup Pico de gallo/salsa
- 2 tablespoons fresh cilantro, chopped
- 1 teaspoon olive oil
- Lime wedges, for garnish
- Hot sauce, for garnish

Instructions:
1. Place a medium skillet over medium flame and heat oil.
2. Stir in onion and cook for 5-8 minutes until crispy-tender.
3. Add rice and black beans in a bowl.
4. Serve with vegetables, cheese, salsa, and cilantro if you are using it.
5. Garnish with lime wedges and hot sauce if you desire.

Nutrition (Per Serving): Calories: 435Fat: 16g Carbohydrates: 60g Protein: 16g Fiber: 10g Sugar: 12gSodium: 584mg

Tip: This is a great recipe to use up your veggie leftovers if you like. If you don't prefer the taste of sharp cheddar cheese, low-fat, you can use mild cheese instead.

75. Healthy Goat Cheese & Arugula Sandwich

Prep Time: 10 minutes
Cook Time: 10 minutes
Servings: 1

Ingredients:
- 2 oz. goat cheese, softened
- 2 oz. pickled beets, sliced
- 2 whole-wheat sandwich bread slices, slightly-toasted
- 1 cup arugula
- 1 tablespoon chopped walnuts, toasted
- 1 tablespoon chives, snipped
- 1 tablespoon fresh dill, chopped
- 1 teaspoon extra-virgin olive oil
- A pinch salt
- Ground pepper, as per taste

Instructions:
1. Add chives, dill, goat cheese, oil, salt and pepper in a bowl and mash it.
2. Take the toast slices and spread the goat cheese mixture on the side of each of them.
3. Add walnuts on top and layer with beets and arugula next.
4. Make the sandwich by topping with the second toast slice, cheese-side facing down and slice it in half.
5. Serve immediately and enjoy with your favorite beverage.

Nutrition (Per Serving): Calories: 414Fat: 24g Carbohydrates: 32g Protein: 18g Fiber: 6g Sugar: 10gSodium: 842mg

Tip: To toast the chopped walnuts, add them to a pan placed over medium-low speed. Continue stirring until golden-brown and fragrant.

76. Creamy Rotisserie Chicken Bowl

Prep Time: 5 minutes
Cook Time: 0 minutes
Servings: 4

Ingredients:
- 2 cups rotisserie chicken, chopped
- ¾ cup celery, chopped
- ⅓ cup lemon-herb aioli
- Cracked black pepper

Instructions:
1. Add chicken and celery in a bowl.
2. Mix in lemon-herb aioli and fold to combine.
3. Season with pepper and serve immediately.

Nutrition (Per Serving): Calories: 230Fat: 16g Carbohydrates: 1g Protein: 21g Fiber: 6g Sugar: 10gSodium: 365mg

Tip: You can find lemon-herb aioli in the condiments section of the grocery store. However, if you cannot find it, use lemon-flavored mayonnaise instead with dill and tarragon to create that taste. You can refrigerate this salad for up to 4 days.

77. Kale & Sun-Dried Tomatoes Snack

Prep Time: 5 minutes
Cook Time: 5 minutes
Servings: 2

Ingredients:
- 1 (10 oz.) package chopped kale
- 1 (15 oz.) can salt-free chickpeas, rinsed
- ¼ cup slivered oil-packed sun-dried tomatoes, and 1 tablespoon oil from the jar
- ⅓ cup water

Instructions:
1. Place a large nonstick skillet over medium flame and heat oil from the sun-dried tomato jar.
2. Stir in kale and cook for 2 minutes until wilted and turns bright green.
3. Pour in water, lower heat to medium-low.
4. Close the lid and cook for 3 additional minutes.
5. Add in chickpeas and sun-dried tomatoes and fold to combine.
6. Let it cook for a minute while stirring until heated through.
7. Remove to a bowl and serve immediately.

Nutrition (Per Serving): Calories: 326Fat: 5g Carbohydrates: 52g Protein: 19g Fiber: 15g Sugar: 5gSodium: 144mg

Tip: If you want to make this more filling, you can add meat or feta, or serve this with rice.

78. Instant Ramen Noodles with Soft-Boiled Egg

Prep Time: 5 minutes
Cook Time: 5 minutes
Servings: 1

Ingredients:
- 1 (3 oz.) package ramen-noodle soup mix
- 1 large soft-boiled egg, halved
- 3 cups water
- 1 cup frozen broccoli
- 1 teaspoon sesame oil, toasted
- ½ teaspoon sesame seeds, toasted

Instructions:
1. Place a medium saucepan over medium flame and boil water.
2. Add in broccoli and cook for 2 minutes.
3. Add in instant ramen noodles and cook for 3 minutes until tender.
4. Drain both the broccoli and noodles well and return to the saucepan.
5. Mix in sesame oil, sesame seeds, and ½ seasoning (save the rest for future use.)
6. Toss well to combine and remove to a bowl.
7. Serve with a soft-boiled egg and enjoy!

Nutrition (Per Serving): Calories: 257Fat: 12g Carbohydrates: 27g Protein: 14g Fiber: 6g Sugar: 4gSodium: 393mg

Tip: To lessen the sodium, pick ramen noodles varieties with less than 600g sodium and be stingy with the packet seasoning

79. Falafel & Tzatziki Tabbouleh Bowls

Prep Time: 5 minutes
Cook Time: 5 minutes
Servings: 4

Ingredients:
- ½ cup tzatziki sauce
- 1 (5 oz.) package salad greens
- 1 (7 oz.) container prepared tabbouleh
- 1 (12 oz.) package frozen falafel

Instructions:
1. Take four small containers and add two tablespoons of tzatziki sauce into each of those containers and refrigerate.
2. Now take four single-person containers with lids and divide tabbouleh among them.
3. Add salad greens on top of each of the containers (a cup per container) and three falafel each.
4. Close the lids and place them in the fridge for up to four days.
5. To serve, first transfer the falafel to a microwave-proof container and heat until heated through.
6. Transfer back to the original container and serve with tzatziki sauce stored in the small containers.

Nutrition (Per Serving): Calories: 416Fat: 26g Carbohydrates: 37g Protein: 11g Fiber: 8g Sugar: 7gSodium: 739mg

Tip: If tabbouleh is unavailable, you can use quinoa for bulger instead.

80. Creamy Cucumber Salad Sandwich

Prep Time: 15 minutes
Cook Time: 0 minutes
Servings: 2

Ingredients:
- 4 whole-grain bread slices, toasted if preferred
- 2 red onions, thinly-sliced
- 1 cup English cucumber, chopped
- ½ cup alfalfa sprouts
- 2 tablespoons low-fat Greek-style yogurt
- 2 tablespoons crumbled feta cheese, low-fat
- 1 tablespoon chopped herbs, like dill/parsley/mint
- ½ teaspoon lemon juice
- ¼ teaspoon lemon zest
- ⅛ teaspoon salt
- ⅛ teaspoon ground pepper

Instructions:
1. Combine cucumber and salt in a medium bowl and set aside for 10 minutes.
2. Meanwhile, mix feta, herbs, yogurt, lemon juice, zest, and pepper in a large bowl.
3. Drain the cucumbers and set on the paper towels to pat dry well.
4. Add them to the yogurt mixture and stir to combine well.
5. Take two bread slices and divide the sprouts among them.
6. Spread the cucumber-yogurt mixture on top of the sprouts, followed with onion slices.
7. Cover with another bread slice to make a sandwich and cut in half.
8. Serve immediately and enjoy with your favorite beverage.

Nutrition (Per Serving): Calories: 293Fat: 6g Carbohydrates: 45g Protein: 16g Fiber: 8g Sugar: 10gSodium: 566

Chapter 11: Dessert Recipes

81. Sweet & Easy Pistachio & Date Bites

Prep Time: 10 minutes
Cook Time: 0 minutes
Servings: 32

Ingredients:
- 2 cups whole dates, pitted
- 1 cup golden raisins
- 1 cup salt-free raw pistachios, shelled
- 1 teaspoon ground fennel seeds
- ¼ teaspoon ground pepper

Instructions:
1. Add all the ingredients in the food processor and process until finely-chopped.
2. Create small 32 balls (a tablespoon each) out of the mixture.
3. You can store them at room temperature in an airtight container for up to 3 hours or refrigerate for snacking.

Nutrition (Per Serving): Calories: 68Fat: 2g Carbohydrates: 13g Protein: 1g Fiber: 1g Sugar: 11gSodium: 1mg

Tip: This is a great healthy snack and you can experiment with it by adding fennel seeds and chia seeds to make this even more filling.

82. Sweet Fig & Honey Yogurt

Prep Time: 5 minutes
Cook Time: 0 minutes
Servings: 1

Ingredients:
- 3 dried figs, sliced
- ⅔ cup low-fat plain yogurt
- 2 teaspoons honey

Instructions:
1. Add yogurt to a bowl.
2. Garnish with figs and honey on top and serve immediately.
3. You can also refrigerate this snack to eat cold later.

Nutrition (Per Serving): Calories: 208Fat: 3g Carbohydrates: 39g Protein: 9g Fiber: 3g Sugar: 35gSodium: 117mg

Tip: You can substitute plain yogurt for Greek-style yogurt if you like. And use fresh figs instead of dried ones if desired.

83. Strawberry & Chocolate Yogurt Bark

Prep Time: 3 hours 10 minutes
Cook Time: 0 minutes
Servings: 32

Ingredients:
- 3 cups plain Greek yogurt, whole-milk
- 1 ½ cups strawberries, sliced
- ¼ cup chocolate chips, mini
- ¼ cup pure maple syrup/honey
- 1 teaspoon vanilla extract

Instructions:
1. Take a large rimmed baking sheet and line it with parchment paper.
2. Combine yogurt, honey or maple syrup, and vanilla extract in a medium bowl.
3. Spread the mixture on the baking sheet into a 10×15-inch rectangle.
4. Add strawberries over the yogurt evenly and sprinkle chocolate chips on top.
5. Put this in the freezer for almost three hours until rigidly firm.
6. Cut or break into 32 pieces before serving.
7. You can freeze this in an airtight container for up to a month wrapped in between parchment paper sheets.

Nutrition (Per Serving): Calories: 34Fat: 1g Carbohydrates: 4g Protein: 2g Fiber: 0g Sugar: 4gSodium: 8mg

Tip: Keep the yogurt spread thick so that it doesn't break or melt easily when cutting into squares or rectangles.

84. Old-Fashioned Apple Crisp Dessert

Prep Time: 20 minutes
Cook Time: 35 minutes
Servings: 8

Ingredients:
- 5 cups baking apples, sliced & peeled
- 2 tablespoons sugar/sugar substitute equivalent
- 1 teaspoon lemon juice
- ½ teaspoon apple pie spice

(Topping)
- ½ cup rolled oats
- ½ cup Frozen & light-whipped dessert topping, thawed
- ¼ cup sugar/sugar substitute equivalent
- 3 tablespoons all-purpose flour
- 3 tablespoons butter
- ¼ teaspoon apple pie spice

Instructions:
1. Start by preheating the oven at 375° F.
2. Combine apples, two tablespoons sugar or sugar equivalent, lemon juice, and ½ teaspoon apple pie spice to create the filling.
3. Take a 2-quart square baking dish and transfer the apple filling into it.
4. Meanwhile, combine oats, ¼ teaspoon apple pie spice, flour, sugar or sugar equivalent in a medium bowl to create the topping.
5. Cut in butter until the topping looks like a coarse crumb.
6. Sprinkle the topping over the filling in the baking dish.
7. Put the baking dish in the oven to bake for 30-35 minutes until the apple is tender and golden-brown.
8. Garnish with whipped cream if you like and serve warm.

Nutrition (Per Serving): Calories: 141Fat: 5g Carbohydrates: 25g Protein: 1g Fiber: 2g Sugar: 17gSodium: 35mg

85. Frozen Chocolate Banana Bites

Prep Time: 2 hours 30 minutes
Cook Time: 0 minutes
Servings: 24

Ingredients:
- 3 large bananas
- ¾ cup vegan chocolate chips
- ¼ cup natural peanut butter, chunky/smooth

Instructions:
1. Peel the bananas and slice each in half lengthwise.
2. Spread peanut butter on each half and close them together to create a banana sandwich.
3. Now slice right rounds or circles from each banana.
4. Line a tray or baking sheet with parchment or butter paper.
5. Arrange the banana bites on the prepared tray and freeze this overnight or for two hours.
6. Meanwhile, add chocolate chips in a microwave-safe bowl and heat them for 1 and a half minutes in 15 seconds increments on high until melted.
7. Take each frozen banana slice and dip half in chocolate.
8. Let it stand until the chocolate is firm.
9. Or you can serve immediately, or freeze it for a few minutes to set the chocolate before serving.

Nutrition (Per Serving): Calories: 58Fat: 3g Carbohydrates: 8g Protein: 1g Fiber: 1g Sugar: 5gSodium: 10mg

Tip: You can store this in a container with a lid for up to a month. Though, eat it only directly from the freezer, or if you have to take it out, then return it to the freezer immediately.

86. Date & Mango Energy Bites

Prep Time: 15 minutes
Cook Time: 0 minutes
Servings: 20

Ingredients:
- 2 cups whole dates, pitted
- 1 cup dried mango/another dried fruit
- 1 cup raw cashews
- ¼ teaspoon salt

Instructions:
1. Add all the ingredients in the food processor and process until finely-chopped.
2. Create 20 balls (two tablespoons each) out of the mixture.
3. You can store them at room temperature in an airtight container or refrigerate for snacking for more than a week.

Nutrition (Per Serving): Calories: 73Fat: 3g Carbohydrates: 11g Protein: 1g Fiber: 1g Sugar: 9gSodium: 35mg

Tip: If cashews are unavailable, you can use any unsalted nuts you like. Same is the case with dried fruit. You can also vacuum seal these in a packet and store them in the freezer for long-term snacking.

87. Banana Flourless Chocolate Chip Muffins

Prep Time: 20 minutes
Cook Time: 20 minutes
Servings: 24

Ingredients:
- 1 ½ cups rolled oats
- 1 cup mashed ripe banana, 2 medium-large sized
- ½ cup mini chocolate chips
- ⅓ cup packed brown sugar
- 2 large eggs
- 3 tablespoons canola oil
- 1 teaspoon baking powder
- 1 teaspoon vanilla extract
- ¼ teaspoon baking soda
- ¼ teaspoon salt

Instructions:
1. Start by preheating the oven at 350 degrees F.
2. Grease a 24-cup mini muffin tray with cooking spray.
3. Finely ground oats in a blender and add baking soda, baking powder, and salt to pulse again.
4. Then add brown sugar, eggs, banana, oil and vanilla extract.
5. Puree until smooth and fold in chocolate chips.
6. Divide the batter among the 24-cup prepared muffin tray.
7. Bake for 15-17 minutes until a toothpick inserted in the middle comes out clean.
8. Place the pan on the wire rack to cool the muffins for 5 minutes.
9. Then remove the muffins from the tray to cool completely.
10. Serve once cool and enjoy with your favorite beverage.

Nutrition (Per Serving): Calories: 78Fat: 4g Carbohydrates: 11g Protein: 1g Fiber: 1g Sugar: 6gSodium: 65mg

88. Quick Peach & Pistachio Toast

Prep Time: 5 minutes
Cook Time: 0 minutes
Servings: 1

Ingredients:
- ½ medium peach, sliced
- 1 whole-wheat bread slice, toasted
- 1 tablespoon part-skim ricotta cheese
- 1 tablespoon pistachios, chopped
- 1 teaspoon honey, divided
- ⅛ teaspoon cinnamon

Instructions:
1. Add cinnamon, ricotta, and ½ teaspoon honey in a bowl.
2. Combine the mixture and spread on the toasted bread slice.
3. Top with peach, sprinkle pistachios and drizzle the remaining ½ teaspoon honey to serve immediately.

Nutrition (Per Serving): Calories: 193Fat: 6g Carbohydrates: 29g Protein: 8g Fiber: 4g Sugar: 14gSodium: 157mg

Tip: Use only fresh peach with this recipe. If you don't have a peach, you can substitute with a fruit you like on toast.

89. Quick & Fresh Pineapple Ice Cream

Prep Time: 5 minutes
Cook Time: 0 minutes
Servings: 6

Ingredients:
- 1 (16 oz.) package frozen pineapple chunks
- 1 cup frozen mango chunks
- 1 tablespoon lemon juice

Instructions
1. Add all the ingredients in the food processor and process until smooth and creamy.
2. In case of frozen ingredients, add ¼ water to the mix if needed for the desired consistency.
3. Serve immediately for the best texture and experience.

Nutrition (Per Serving): Calories: 55Fat: 0g Carbohydrates: 14g Protein: 1g Fiber: 2g Sugar: 11gSodium: 1mg

Tip: You can use fresh mango but first peel, seed and cut it into chunks before use. And you can substitute lemon juice with lime juice in case of unavailability.

90. Easy Watermelon Sherbet

Prep Time: 8 hours 10 minutes
Cook Time: 0 minutes
Servings: 12

Ingredients:
- 1 (14 oz.) can sweetened condensed milk
- 6 ¼ cups watermelon, cubed & seedless
- ⅓ cup lime juice
- ¼ teaspoon salt

Instructions:
1. Take a large rimmed baking sheet and place the watermelon on it.
2. Freeze it for 4 hours or overnight until frozen.
3. Add all the ingredients including the frozen watermelon cubes in the food processor.
4. Work in batches if you have to and puree the mixture for 2-3 minutes until smooth.
5. Transfer the puree to a large sealable container, cover and freeze for 4 hours or overnight until set.
6. Serve immediately and enjoy!

Nutrition (Per Serving): Calories: 132Fat: 3g Carbohydrates: 25g Protein: 3g Fiber: 0g Sugar: 23gSodium: 91mg

Tip: You can freeze this for up to a week.

Chapter 12: Sauces, Condiments & Dressing

91. Spinach & Walnut Pesto

Prep Time: 10 minutes
Cook Time: 5 minutes
Servings: 8

Ingredients:
- 1 oz. Parmesan cheese, low-fat, grated
- 1 small garlic clove, chopped
- 4 cups fresh spinach
- ¼ cup walnuts, toasted
- 3 tablespoons olive oil
- 2 tablespoons warm water
- 2 teaspoons fresh lemon juice
- ¼ teaspoon crushed red pepper

Instructions:
1. Add all the ingredients except olive oil and warm in the food processor.
2. Process everything until finely-chopped.
3. Meanwhile, gradually add olive oil through the food chute to the mix with the food processor on.
4. Pour in warm water and process until well blended.

Nutrition (Per Serving): Calories: 85Fat: 8g Carbohydrates: 2g Protein: 2g Fiber: 1g Sugar: 11gSodium: 76mg

Tip: To toast the walnuts, place a skillet over medium heat and stir in the walnuts for 5 minutes until fragrant and golden-brown.

92. Italian Olive Dressing

Prep Time: 10 minutes
Cook Time: 5 minutes
Servings: 6

Ingredients:
- ⅓ cup extra-virgin olive oil
- 3 tablespoons red-wine vinegar
- 2 tablespoons mayonnaise
- 1 teaspoon sugar
- 1 teaspoon Dijon mustard
- ¾ teaspoon Italian seasoning
- ¼ teaspoon salt
- ¼ teaspoon garlic powder
- ¼ teaspoon ground pepper

Instructions:
1. Add all the ingredients in a jar container in an airtight sealing lid.
2. Seal the lid and shake to well combine.

Nutrition (Per Serving): Calories: 149Fat: 18g Carbohydrates: 1g Protein: 9g Fiber: 0g Sugar: 1gSodium: 155mg

93. Homemade Garlic Aioli

Prep Time: 10 minutes
Cook Time: 0 minutes
Servings: 20

Ingredients:
- 1 large egg yolk, at room temperature
- 4 garlic cloves, finely-chopped
- ½ cup canola oil
- ½ cup extra-virgin olive oil
- 2 teaspoons fresh lemon juice
- ¼ teaspoon salt

Instructions:
1. Finely chop garlic onto a cutting board and season with salt.
2. Take a chef's knife and use its flat side to crush the garlic until it turns into a smooth paste.
3. Transfer it to a large bowl and set aside.
4. Meanwhile, whisk egg yolk and lemon juice in another bowl until smooth.

5. Gradually add canola oil into the mix drop by drop while whisking continuously.
6. As soon as the mixture starts to thicken and emulsify, increase the canola oil ratio until it drops like a steady, thin stream and don't stop whisking.
7. Then slowly pour in olive oil while whisking until aioli begins to get thick, creamy and smooth.
8. You can serve this sauce for dipping vegetables, French fries, or consume as a sandwich spread.

Nutrition (Per Serving): Calories: 101Fat: 11g Carbohydrates: 0g Protein: 0g Fiber: 0g Sugar: 0gSodium: 30mg

94. Easy & Creamy Chipotle Sauce

Prep Time: 10 minutes
Cook Time: 0 minutes
Servings: 10

Ingredients:
- 1 garlic clove
- ½ teaspoon salt
- ⅓ cup sour cream
- ¼ teaspoon ground cumin
- 1 teaspoon honey, if desired
- 1 tablespoon fresh lime juice
- ¼ cup packed fresh cilantro leaves & tender stems
- ½ cup whole-milk plain strained yogurt, Greek-style
- 3 canned chipotle peppers in adobo + 1 tablespoon adobo sauce

Instructions:
1. Add all the ingredients in the food processor.
2. Process until creamy and very smooth and the cilantro leaves are finely-chopped.
3. This will take a minute or two to get to your desired consistency.
4. You can refrigerate this in an airtight container for up to a week.

5. You can also serve this with French fries, pasta, fritters or fresh crunchy veggies.

Nutrition (Per Serving): Calories: 28Fat: 2g Carbohydrates: 1g Protein: 2g Fiber: 0g Sugar: 2gSodium: 144mg

Tip: Honey is an optional ingredient but it helps to balance the heat of the chipotle sauce

95. Easy White Wine Sauce

Prep Time: 5 minutes
Cook Time: 7 minutes
Servings: 1

Ingredients:
- ½ cup fat-free & low-sodium chicken broth
- ⅓ cup onion, finely-chopped
- ¼ cup dry white wine
- 2 tablespoons butter
- 2 tablespoons white wine vinegar
- 2 teaspoons fresh chives, finely-chopped
- Cooking spray, as needed

Instructions:
1. Place a skillet over medium-high heat and grease with cooking spray.
2. Stir finely-chopped onion in the pan and sauté for two minutes.
3. Add in dry white wine, broth, and white wine vinegar.
4. Stir and bring it to a boil and cook for 5 minutes until the mixture is reduced to ¼ cup.
5. Take the skillet off from heat and stir in butter and fresh chives.
6. Serve the sauce with grilled chicken breast or pan-seared fish.

Nutrition (Per Serving): Calories: 59Fat: 6g Carbohydrates: 2g Protein: 0g Fiber: 0g Sugar: 0gSodium: 90mg

Tip: If chicken broth is not available, you can use low-sodium vegetable broth instead.

96. Lemon & Garlic Vinaigrette

Prep Time: 5 minutes
Cook Time: 7 minutes
Servings: 1

Ingredients:
- 1 garlic clove, grated
- ¾ cup extra-virgin olive oil
- 5 tablespoons red wine vinegar
- 3 tablespoons lemon juice
- 1 ½ tablespoons Dijon mustard
- ¾ teaspoon salt
- Ground pepper, as per taste

Instructions:
1. Add all the ingredients in a jar container in an airtight sealing lid.
2. Seal the lid and shake to well combine.
3. Use this as a salad dressing!

Nutrition (Per Serving): Calories: 130Fat: 14g Carbohydrates: 0g Protein: 0g Fiber: 0g Sugar: 0gSodium: 191mg

Tip: You can store this in the refrigerator for up to 1 week. Shake it before use every time!

97. Sweet Tart Balsamic Marinade

Prep Time: 2 minutes
Cook Time: 5 minutes
Servings: 4

Ingredients:
- 2 garlic cloves, minced
- ¼ cup balsamic vinegar
- ¼ cup extra virgin olive oil
- 1 tablespoon Italian seasoning
- 1 teaspoon salt
- ½ teaspoon freshly ground pepper

Instructions:
1. Whisk all the ingredients in a bowl until melded together well.
2. This is the perfect marinade for anything you want to grill.

Nutrition (Per Serving): Calories: 24Fat: 2g Carbohydrates: 1g Protein: 0g Fiber: 0g Sugar: 0gSodium: 98mg

Tip: You can also use a large shallot instead of two garlic cloves instead in case of availability issues.

98. Quick & Easy Cucumber Pickles

Prep Time: 4 days
Cook Time: 2 minutes
Servings: 7 cups

Ingredients:
- 6 cups (2 pounds) pickling cucumbers, thinly-sliced
- 2 cups onion, thinly-sliced
- 1 ½ cups white vinegar
- 4 garlic cloves, thinly-sliced
- ¾ cup sugar
- ¾ teaspoon salt
- ½ teaspoon mustard seeds
- ½ teaspoon celery seeds
- ½ teaspoon ground turmeric
- ½ teaspoon crushed red pepper
- ¼ teaspoon freshly ground black pepper

Instructions:
1. Put 3 cups of cucumber in a bowl and top with 1 cup onion.
2. Repeat the same with the remaining cups of cucumber and onion.
3. Combine the remaining ingredients in a small saucepan.
4. Stir thoroughly and place it on the stove over medium flame.
5. Bring to a bowl and let it cook for a minute.

6. Pour this over the cucumber and onion mixture and let it cool.
7. Cover and refrigerate for four days.
8. Serve as a side dish with any main dish whenever you like.

Nutrition (Per Serving): Calories: 28Fat: 0g Carbohydrates: 7g Protein: 0g Fiber: 0g Sugar: 0gSodium: 64mg

Tip: You can store these cucumber pickles in the refrigerator for up to a month. It's best to store it in an airtight sanitized jar.

99. Roasted Garlic Parmesan Cream Sauce

Prep Time: 15 minutes
Cook Time: 15 minutes
Servings: 8

Ingredients:
- 6 garlic cloves, unpeeled
- 1 tablespoon butter
- 2 tablespoons all-purpose flour
- 1 cup low-fat milk, warm
- ½ cup Parmesan cheese, low-fat, grated
- ¼ teaspoon salt
- ⅛ teaspoon ground pepper

Instructions:
1. Place a small cast-iron skillet on medium flame and cook garlic.
2. Stir constantly and cook for 12-15 minutes until the garlic turns brown and soft from inside.
3. Remove to a cutting board and cool it.
4. Once cool, peel the cloves and mash them into a smooth paste.
5. Meanwhile, place a medium saucepan over medium flame and stir in butter until melted.
6. Whisk in flour in the butter until well combined.
7. Then slowly add in milk while whisking constantly so there are no lumps.
8. Cook and stir this for 6-8 minutes until thickened.
9. Lower the heat to low flame and mix in the garlic paste with Parmesan, salt and pepper.
10. Cook and whisk constantly for a minute until the cheese has melted and everything is combined well.

Nutrition (Per Serving): Calories: 57Fat: 3g Carbohydrates: 5g Protein: 3g Fiber: 0g Sugar: 2gSodium: 164mg

Tip: Serve with pasta mixed with this sauce or use it as a pizza sauce.

100. Homemade Rosemary & Red Wine Marinade

Prep Time: 10 minutes
Cook Time: 0 minutes
Servings: 1

Ingredients:
- 4 garlic cloves, minced
- ½ cup red wine vinegar
- ⅓ cup dry red wine
- 2 tablespoons fresh rosemary, chopped
- 1 tablespoon extra-virgin olive oil
- 1 teaspoon salt
- ½ teaspoon freshly ground pepper

Instructions:
1. Whisk all the ingredients in a bowl until melded together well.
2. This is the perfect marinade for beef, chicken thighs, or lamb.
3. Use half cup for marinating and half for basting.

Nutrition (Per Serving): Calories: 24Fat: 2g Carbohydrates: 1g Protein: 0g Fiber: 0g Sugar: 0gSodium: 98mg

Chapter 13: Quick & Easy Meal

101. Easy Pesto Ravioli

Prep Time: 5 minutes
Cook Time: 10 minutes
Servings: 4

Ingredients:
- 2 (8 oz.) packages frozen/refrigerated cheese ravioli
- 1 5 oz. package baby spinach
- 1-pint grape tomatoes
- ⅓ cup pesto
- 1 tablespoon olive oil

Instructions:
1. Place a large pot of water over medium-high flame and bring it to a boil.
2. Cook the ravioli according to the package directions, drain well and put aside.
3. Next, place a nonstick skillet over medium flame and heat oil.
4. Stir in tomatoes and sauté for 4-5 minutes until they break down.
5. Stir in spinach and cook for 2 minutes until wilted.
6. Stir in the pesto and ravioli and combine well.
7. Remove to serving bowls and serve immediately!

Nutrition (Per Serving): Calories: 361Fat: 19g Carbohydrates: 35g Protein: 14g Fiber: 4g Sugar: 6gSodium: 407mg

Tip: You can add finely chopped onion and garlic into the mix to enhance the flavor. Also, if you can't find ravioli, you can substitute it with other pasta varieties.

102. Buttered & Seared Scallops

Prep Time: 5 minutes
Cook Time: 5 minutes
Servings: 4

Ingredients:
- 1 pound (16) sea scallops, hard-side-muscle-removed & pat-dry
- 3 tablespoons unsalted butter, divided
- 1 tablespoon chopped fresh herbs, like tarragon/sage/parsley
- 1 tablespoon lemon juice
- ¼ teaspoon salt
- ¼ teaspoon ground pepper

Instructions:
1. Place a large skillet over medium flame and heat a tablespoon of butter.
2. Season scallops with salt and pepper and cook for 3 minutes until golden-brown from the bottom.
3. Flip the scallops and stir in the herbs and remaining butter.
4. Continue cooking for 2-3 minutes while spooning the buttery gravy over the scallops until they are cooked through and browned from the bottom.
5. Remove the pan from heat and mix in lemon juice.
6. Divide the scallops among serving plates and spoon the gravy on top.

Nutrition (Per Serving): Calories: 157Fat: 9g Carbohydrates: 4g Protein: 14g Fiber: 0g Sugar: 0gSodium: 591mg

Tip: Make sure to buy dry sea scallops for this recipe that have not been treated with STP "sodium tripolyphosphate." Those treated with this chemical (wet scallops) don't brown as well and aren't as flavorful either.

103. Quick Black Bean Quesadillas

Prep Time: 5 minutes
Cook Time: 10 minutes
Servings: 4

Ingredients:
- 1 (15 oz.) can black beans, rinsed
- 4 (8 inch) whole wheat tortillas
- 1 ripe avocado, diced
- ½ cup shredded Monterey Jack cheese, pepper Jack favorably
- ½ cup prepared fresh salsa, divided
- 2 teaspoons canola oil, divided

Instructions:
1. Place a large nonstick skillet over medium flame and heat a teaspoon of oil.
2. But before that, prepare quesadillas by combining ¼ cup salsa, black beans, and cheese in a medium bowl.
3. Spread ½ cup filling on one side of each tortilla and cover with the other half into a fold and flatten with light pressure.
4. Place 2 folded quesadillas on the hot pan and cook both sides for 2 minutes each until toasted and golden-brown.
5. Remove to a cutting board and cover with foil to keep warm.
6. Repeat the same process with the remaining quesadillas.
7. Serve them with the remaining salsa and avocado.

Nutrition (Per Serving): Calories: 378Fat: 16g Carbohydrates: 45g Protein: 13g Fiber: 10g Sugar: 6gSodium: 608mg

Tip: The prepared salsa can be found in a supermarket's refrigerator section near other dips and sauces.

104. Stuffed Potatoes & Salsa

Prep Time: 10 minutes
Cook Time: 15 minutes
Servings: 4

Ingredients:
- 1 (15 oz.) can pinto beans, rinsed, warmed, & slightly-mashed
- 4 medium Yukon potatoes
- 1 ripe avocado, sliced
- ½ cup fresh salsa
- 4 teaspoons pickled jalapeños, chopped

Instructions:
1. Start by preheating the oven at 425 degrees F.
2. Use a fork to pierce the potatoes all over.
3. Microwave them for 20 minutes, turning once or twice after few minutes, until they are soft.
4. Or bake in the oven for 45 minutes until tender and toasted.
5. Remove to a clean cutting board and let them cool for a bit.
6. Handle the potatoes with a kitchen towel to protect your handles and cut them enough lengthwise just to open the potato or create a pocket but not cut all the way through.
7. Pinch the ends to reveal the flesh and fill with salsa, avocado, jalapenos and beans.
8. Remove to serving plates to serve immediately!

Nutrition (Per Serving): Calories: 324Fat: 8g Carbohydrates: 57g Protein: 9g Fiber: 11g Sugar: 5gSodium: 422mg

Tip: You can add chopped cilantro on top for added taste and garnish.

105. Chicken & Strawberry Poppy Seed Salad

Prep Time: 10 minutes
Cook Time: 0 minutes
Servings: 2

Ingredients:
- 4 large strawberries, hulled & sliced
- 4 cups mixed salad greens
- 1 cup diced cooked chicken
- ¼ cup (1 oz.) goat cheese, crumbled
- ¼ cup chopped toasted pecans, if desired
- 3 tablespoons low-sodium & low-added-sugar poppy seed dressing

Instructions:
1. Combine all the ingredients except the dressing in a large bowl.
2. Add in the dressing and toss to coat.
3. Serve with the pecans sprinkled on top if you like.

Nutrition (Per Serving): Calories: 265Fat: 15g Carbohydrates: 15g Protein: 18g Fiber: 3g Sugar: 9gSodium: 423mg

Tip: If poppy seed dressing is unavailable, use other salad dressing preferably with low-sodium and low added-sugar.

106. Butternut Squash Soup with Halloumi

Prep Time: 10 minutes
Cook Time: 5 minutes
Servings: 4

Ingredients:
- 1 (32 oz.) carton low-sodium butternut squash soup
- 4 oz. halloumi cheese, cut-into-½ inch-pieces
- 1 teaspoon olive oil
- 1 teaspoon curry powder
- 4 teaspoons toasted pepitas

Instructions:
1. Place a large pan over medium flame and heat the soup according to the package directions.
2. Mix in the curry powder and lower the heat to a simmer for 3 minutes.
3. Meanwhile, dry the cheese slices with a paper towel.
4. Brush each side of cheese slices with oil and sear in a heavy-bottomed pan over medium flame for 1-2 minutes each side until golden-brown.
5. Ladle out the soup into serving bowls and top with cheese and pepitas.

Nutrition (Per Serving): Calories: 203Fat: 13g Carbohydrates: 17g Protein: 9g Fiber: 3g Sugar: 4gSodium: 564mg

Tip: To make the soup more filling, eat it with whole wheat pita bread!

107. Teriyaki Edamame Stir Fry

Prep Time: 5 minutes
Cook Time: 5 minutes
Servings: 2

Ingredients:
- 1 (8 oz.) bag tricolor coleslaw mix
- 2 cups shelled edamame, thaw if frozen
- ¼ cup low-sodium teriyaki sauce
- 1 tablespoon olive oil

Instructions:
1. Place a large nonstick skillet over medium flame and heat oil.
2. Stir in coleslaw mix and sauté for 2 minutes until the cabbage turns soft.
3. Add in teriyaki sauce and edamame, stir and cook until heated through.
4. Cook for a minute more until the sauce thickens.
5. Remove to a serving bowl and serve immediately!

Nutrition (Per Serving): Calories: 249Fat: 12g Carbohydrates: 21g Protein: 17g Fiber: 8g Sugar: 8gSodium: 670mg

Tip: Serve this with whole wheat pita bread to make it more filling.

108. Tex-Mex Black Beans & Fajita

Prep Time: 5 minutes
Cook Time: 10 minutes
Servings: 2

Ingredients:
- 1 (12 oz.) package sliced fajita vegetables like onions
- 1 oz. (¼ cup) coarsely-shredded Cheddar cheese, low-fat, optional
- 1 (15 oz.) can salt-free black beans, rinsed
- 1 tablespoon olive oil
- ½ teaspoon salt-free Southwest-style seasoning blend
- ¼ teaspoon salt

Instructions:
1. Place a large skillet over medium heat and heat oil.
2. Sauté fajita vegetables for 10 minutes until tender.
3. Stir in black beans with seasoning and salt and cook for a minute until heated through.
4. Transfer the stir fry equally into two bowls and top with cheese if using to serve immediately.

Nutrition (Per Serving): Calories: 310Fat: 8g Carbohydrates: 47g Protein: 14g Fiber: 17g Sugar: 8gSodium: 602mg

Tip: You can make this even more fulfilling by adding avocado and serving with brown rice.

109. Asparagus & Cauliflower Gnocchi

Prep Time: 10 minutes
Cook Time: 10 minutes
Servings: 2

Ingredients:
- 1 (10 oz.) bag frozen cauliflower gnocchi
- 8 oz. asparagus spears, trimmed
- ⅓ cup basil pesto
- 1 tablespoon olive oil

Instructions:
1. Place a large nonstick skillet over medium flame and heat oil.
2. Stir in gnocchi and cook for 6-8 minutes until heated through and golden-brown.
3. Add ¼ inch water in a microwave-safe bowl and add in asparagus.
4. Cover tightly and microwave for 2 minutes until crispy-tender and vivid green.
5. Drain well and chop into 1-inch pieces and add to the gnocchi along with pesto.
6. Toss to combine and serve immediately!

Nutrition (Per Serving): Calories: 404Fat: 27g Carbohydrates: 29g Protein: 9g Fiber: 9g Sugar: 5gSodium: 256mg

Tip: If asparagus isn't available, substitute it with green beans or peas.

110. Stuffed Sweet Potatoes

Prep Time: 10 minutes
Cook Time: 10 minutes
Servings: 4

Ingredients:
- 4 (8 oz. each) medium sweet potatoes
- 8 oz. cooked chicken, chopped & warmed
- 1 ½ cups cooked cauliflower, chopped
- ½ cup Madras curry sauce
- 4 teaspoons fresh cilantro, chopped

Instructions:
1. Start by preheating the oven at 425 degrees F.
2. Use a fork to pierce the potatoes all over.
3. Microwave them for 20 minutes, turning once or twice after few minutes, until they are soft.
4. Or bake in the oven for 45 minutes to an hour until tender and toasted.
5. Remove to a clean cutting board and let them cool for a bit.
6. Handle the potatoes with a kitchen towel to protect your handles and cut them enough lengthwise just to open the potato or create a pocket but not cut all the way through.
7. Pinch the ends to reveal the flesh and fill with curry sauce, chicken, and cilantro
8. Remove to serving plates and serve immediately!

Nutrition (Per Serving): Calories: 257Fat: 5g Carbohydrates: 30g Protein: 22g Fiber: 5g Sugar: 11gSodium: 240mg

Tip: If curry sauce is unavailable, look into Thai red curry pasta or Tikka masala pasta instead.

Chapter 14: Meals on a Budget

111. Steamed Green Beans

Prep Time: 5 minutes
Cook Time: 5 minutes
Servings: 4

Ingredients:
- 1 pound trimmed green beans

Instructions:
1. Place a large saucepan with a fitted steamer basket on medium-high flame.
2. Boil an inch of water in the saucepan and add in the green beans.
3. Steam them covered for 5-7 minutes until crispy-tender.
4. Use them as a side dish, add in a salad or serve with mashed potatoes.

Nutrition (Per Serving): Calories: 27Fat: 0g Carbohydrates: 7g Protein: 1g Fiber: 4g Sugar: 3gSodium: 407mg

Tip: To trim the green beans, line them up on a cutting board and cut off their stem ends to save time.

112. Brown Rice & Black Beans Bowl

Prep Time: 10 minutes
Cook Time: 10 minutes
Servings: 1

Ingredients:
- 1 oz. (¼ cup) sharp Cheddar cheese, low-fat, shredded
- ½ red onion, sliced
- ½ cup brown rice, cooked
- ¼ cup canned black beans, rinsed
- ¼ cup Pico de gallo/salsa
- 1 teaspoon olive oil
- 2 tablespoons chopped fresh cilantro, for garnish
- Lime wedges, for garnish
- Hot sauce, for garnish

Instructions:
1. Place a medium skillet over medium flame and heat oil.
2. Stir in onion and sauté for 5-8 minutes until crispy-tender.
3. Add rice and black beans in a bowl followed with onion, cheese, Pico de gallo or salsa.
4. Serve immediately, garnished with cilantro, lime wedges and hot sauce if you like.

Nutrition (Per Serving): Calories: 435Fat: 16g Carbohydrates: 60g Protein: 16g Fiber: 10g Sugar: 12gSodium: 584mg

Tip: You can be experimental with this recipe and use leftovers with this dish.

113. Stuffed Avocado with Salmon

Prep Time: 15 minutes
Cook Time: 0 minutes
Servings: 4

Ingredients:
- 2 (5 oz.) cans drained & flaked salmon, skin-&-bones-cut-off
- 2 avocados
- ½ cup celery, diced
- ½ cup nonfat plain Greek yogurt
- 2 tablespoons fresh parsley, chopped
- 1 tablespoon lime juice
- 2 teaspoons mayonnaise
- 1 teaspoon Dijon mustard
- ⅛ teaspoon salt
- ⅛ teaspoon ground pepper
- Chopped chives, for garnish

Instructions:
1. Combine all the ingredients in a medium bowl except avocado.
2. Cut avocados in half lengthwise and discard the pits.
3. Scoop a tablespoon of flesh from each avocado half and dump it into a separate bowl.
4. Mix the avocado flesh by first mashing it and then adding to combine in the salmon mixture.
5. Stuff each avocado half with ¼ cup salmon mixture.
6. Sprinkle chopped chives if you like on top and serve immediately.

Nutrition (Per Serving): Calories: 293Fat: 20g Carbohydrates: 11g Protein: 23g Fiber: 7g Sugar: 2gSodium: 400mg

Tip: You can use the leftovers with whole wheat toast in breakfast. You can also add cucumber and chopped tomato to the mixture to make it more filling.

114. Healthy Kale & Banana Smoothie

Prep Time: 10 minutes
Cook Time: 0 minutes
Servings: 1

Ingredients:
- 1 ½ cups baby kale
- 1 cup low-fat milk/non-dairy milk
- 1 small banana, sliced
- 6 ice cubes
- 2 teaspoons honey

Instructions:
1. Add all the ingredients in the blender and blend on medium-low speed.
2. Use the tamper as needed and increase the speed to medium-high until very smooth.
3. Pour the smoothie into a glass and serve immediately.

Nutrition (Per Serving): Calories: 266Fat: 5g Carbohydrates: 48g Protein: 10g Fiber: 4g Sugar: 36gSodium: 129mg

Tip: You can use cow milk for a thicker consistency. Oat milk for added sweetness and nut milk for higher protein count.

115. Edamame & Beets Salad

Prep Time: 15 minutes
Cook Time: 0 minutes
Servings: 1

Ingredients:
- 2 cups mixed salad greens
- 1 cup shelled edamame, thawed
- ½ cup medium raw beet, peeled & shredded
- 2 tablespoons red wine vinegar
- 1 tablespoon fresh cilantro, chopped
- 1 tablespoon extra-virgin olive oil
- ⅛ teaspoon salt
- Freshly ground pepper, as per taste

Instructions:
1. Mix together vinegar, oil, cilantro, salt and pepper in a small bowl.
2. Arrange all the greens with raw beet in a bowl or platter and add the dressing.
3. Toss to combine until everything is melded together.
4. Serve immensely as a side or a main.

Nutrition (Per Serving): Calories: 356Fat: 26g Carbohydrates: 21g Protein: 21g Fiber: 11g Sugar: 7gSodium: 263mg

Tip: You can refrigerate the salad and dressing separately and store this for up to two days. When making the salad, shake the dressing before use and drizzle it in the salad for fresh taste.

116. Indian Paneer Saag

Prep Time: 25 minutes
Cook Time: 0 minutes
Servings: 4

Ingredients:
- 20 oz. finely-chopped frozen spinach, thawed
- 8 oz. paneer cheese, ½-inch-cubes
- 2 cups low-fat plain yogurt
- 1 small onion, finely chopped
- 1 garlic clove, minced
- 2 tablespoons extra-virgin olive oil, divided
- 1 tablespoon fresh ginger, minced
- 2 teaspoons garam masala
- 1 teaspoon ground cumin
- ¾ teaspoon salt
- ¼ teaspoon ground turmeric
- 1 finely-chopped jalapeño pepper, optional

Instructions:
1. Place a nonstick skillet over medium flame and heat a tablespoon oil.
2. Meanwhile, add paneer in a medium bowl with turmeric and toss to coat.
3. Add the paneer in the hot skillet and cook both sides for 5 minutes until browned, flipping only once.
4. Remove to a plate and set aside.
5. Heat the remaining oil in the same skillet and add in onion and jalapeno.
6. Sauté for 7-8 minutes until golden-brown and fragrant.
7. If the skillet feels a little dry during cooking, add in a little water like two tablespoons.
8. Now add in ginger, garam masala, garlic, and cumin.
9. Stir for 30 seconds and then add spinach and salt.
10. Cook for 3 minutes and remove from heat.
11. Then stir in yogurt and paneer.
12. Serve immediately and enjoy!

Nutrition (Per Serving): Calories: 382Fat: 24g Carbohydrates: 19g Protein: 25g Fiber: 5g Sugar: 11gSodium: 641mg

Tip: You can serve this dish with brown rice for a more fulfilling meal.

117. Tuna with Chickpea Salad

Prep Time: 20 minutes
Cook Time: 0 minutes
Servings: 4

Ingredients:
- 1 (15 oz.) can salt-free chickpeas, rinsed
- 1 (6.7 oz.) jar oil-packed tuna, drained
- 3 cups baby spinach
- 1 cup cherry tomatoes, halved
- 1 cup English cucumber, thinly-sliced
- ½ cup crumbled feta cheese, low-fat
- 3 tablespoons extra-virgin olive oil
- 2 tablespoons fresh dill, chopped
- 2 tablespoons lemon juice
- 1 tablespoon nonpareil capers, rinsed & chopped
- 1 tablespoon shallot, finely-chopped
- ¼ teaspoon salt
- ¼ teaspoon ground pepper

Instructions:
1. Mix capers, shallot, lemon juice, salt and pepper in a large bowl and set aside for 5 minutes.
2. Next combine tuna, chickpeas, tomatoes, feta, cucumber and dill in a separate large bowl and toss.
3. Whisk oil into the capers mixture until well combined and add 5 tablespoons to the chickpea bowl.
4. Toss to combine and add spinach to the dressing bowl to combine.
5. Serve spinach equally among 4 plates and top with the chickpea mixture.

Nutrition (Per Serving): Calories: 357Fat: 19g Carbohydrates: 23g Protein: 21g Fiber: 6g Sugar: 3gSodium: 555mg

Tip: You can store this salad separately in the refrigerator for up to a day. Shake the dressing before adding it to the salad.

118. Sweet Potato & Quinoa Chili

Prep Time: 15 minutes
Cook Time: 15 minutes
Servings: 5

Ingredients:
- 1 (15 oz.) can salt-free pinto beans, rinsed
- 2 (12 oz.) sweet potatoes, peeled & cut-into-½-inch-pieces
- 1 (10 oz.) can salt-free tomatoes with green chiles, diced
- 1 (4 oz.) can green chiles, diced
- 4 cups unsalted vegetable broth
- 2 cups water, divided
- 1 cup white/multicolored quinoa, uncooked
- 4 large garlic cloves, chopped
- 1 bell pepper, diced
- 1 medium yellow onion, diced
- 1 tablespoon extra-virgin olive oil
- 1 tablespoon chili powder
- 2 teaspoons ground cumin
- ½ teaspoon salt
- Sliced jalapeño peppers, for garnish
- Yogurt, for garnish
- Cilantro, for garnish

Instructions:
1. Place a large pot over medium-high flame and heat oil.
2. Stir in sweet potatoes and cook for 6-7 minutes until soft and lightly charred.
3. Stir in onions and bell pepper and cook for 3 minutes until fragrant.
4. Stir in garlic, cumin, and chili powder for 30 seconds.
5. Pour in broth and add tomatoes, green chiles, and a cup of water.
6. Close the lid, increase the flame to high and bring it to a boil.
7. Add in quinoa, beans and salt while stirring.
8. Lower the heat to a simmer and cover the lid.
9. Cook and stir for 15 minutes until the quinoa is tender and add the remaining cup of water during the final 3 minutes of cooking.
10. Ladle out the chili into serving plates and garnish with yogurt, jalapeno peppers, and cilantro.

Nutrition (Per Serving): Calories: 346Fat: 6g Carbohydrates: 63g Protein: 12g Fiber: 11g Sugar: 11gSodium: 703mg

Tip: You can store the chili for up to 5 days in an airtight container in the fridge. Or for more than 2 months in the freezer.

119. Orange Tofu with Chipotle

Prep Time: 15 minutes
Cook Time: 15 minutes
Servings: 4

Ingredients:
- 1 (14 oz.) package extra-firm water-packed tofu
- 6 cups broccoli florets
- 1 cup orange juice
- ½ cup fresh cilantro, chopped
- 3 tablespoons canola oil, divided
- 1 tablespoon minced chipotle in adobo, seeded if preferred
- ½ teaspoon salt, divided

Instructions:
1. Place a large nonstick skillet over medium-high flame and heat two tablespoons oil.
2. Meanwhile, drain tofu and pat dry with kitchen towels.
3. Cut it into ½-¾ inches cubes and season all over with salt.
4. Add to the hot pan and cook it in a single layer for 7-9 minutes while stirring until golden-brown.
5. Remove to a plate and set aside.
6. Heat the remaining oil in the skillet and add broccoli with the remaining salt.
7. Cook for a minute while stirring until bright green and add orange juice.
8. Next add in chipotle and stir and cook for 2-3 minutes until broccoli gets tender.
9. Add the tofu to the pan and toss it gently with the broccoli until heated through for a minute or two.
10. Remove to a serving bowl and garnish with cilantro on top.

Nutrition (Per Serving): Calories: 242Fat: 17g Carbohydrates: 14g Protein: 14g Fiber: 4g Sugar: 6gSodium: 337mg

Tip: Adobo sauce with minced chipotle can be found in large markets under Mexican foods. For added favor, you can add a tablespoon or two of soy sauce.

120. Quick Vegetarian Chili

Prep Time: 15 minutes
Cook Time: 15 minutes
Servings: 4

Ingredients:
- 2 (15 oz.) cans reduced-sodium black beans, rinsed
- 1 (14 oz.) can tomatoes, diced
- 4 garlic cloves, chopped
- ½ cup shredded cheese, like Cheddar/pepper Jack
- ¾ cup white onion, finely-chopped
- ¼ cup water
- 2 tablespoons chili powder
- 1 tablespoon canola oil
- 1 tablespoon ground cumin
- 2 teaspoons dried oregano
- 1 teaspoon ground coriander

Instructions:
1. Place a large saucepan over medium-high flame and heat oil.
2. Sauté onion and garlic for 8 minutes until tender.
3. Stir in cumin, oregano, chilli powder, and coriander for 30 seconds.
4. Add in tomatoes and their juice, beans, water and let it simmer for 5 minutes.
5. Remove to serving plates and garnish with cheese on top.

Nutrition (Per Serving): Calories: 311Fat: 11g Carbohydrates: 39g Protein: 16g Fiber: 14g Sugar: 4gSodium: 434mg

Tip: You can refrigerate this without cheese for up to 3 days or store it in the freezer for up to 3 months. Only sprinkle cheese before serving.

121. Vegetarian Fried Rice

Prep Time: 10 minutes
Cook Time: 15 minutes
Servings: 4

Ingredients:
- 4 large eggs, lightly-whisked
- 2 sliced scallions with greens & whites separated, divided
- 4 cups cauliflower rice
- ½ cup unsalted peanuts
- 2 tablespoons peanut oil, divided
- 2 tablespoons chile-garlic sauce, like sambal Oelek
- 1 tablespoon fresh ginger, minced
- 2 teaspoons low-sodium soy sauce/tamari

Instructions:
1. Place a large nonstick skillet over medium-high flame and heat a tablespoon of oil.
2. Add eggs and cook for 2 minutes, tilting the pan and lifting the edges using a spatula so that the uncooked egg can flow to the bottom.
3. Once the egg from the bottom is set, flip and continue cooking the other side until firm for 30 seconds more.
4. Remove to a cutting board and cut into bite-sized strips.
5. Heat the remaining oil in the skillet over medium-high flame.
6. Add in cauliflower rice, scallion whites, ginger.
7. Stir and cook for 5 minutes until cauliflower rice starts to brown and get soft.
8. Stir in soy sauce/tamari, chile-garlic sauce, peanuts, and the eggs.
9. Stir for 30 seconds until heated through and combined well.
10. Remove to a serving bowl and garnish with green scallions.

Nutrition (Per Serving): Calories: 291Fat: 21g Carbohydrates: 13g Protein: 14g Fiber: 4g Sugar: 5gSodium: 441mg

Tip: Prepared cauliflower rice or cauliflower crumbles can be found in the supermarket under the prepared vegetables section. Though, to make your own cauliflower rice, pulse cauliflower florets in a food processor until they turn into rice-like granules. A single 2-pound cauliflower head makes 4 cups cauliflower rice.

122. Vegetables & Hummus Sandwich

Prep Time: 10 minutes
Cook Time: 0 minutes
Servings: 1

Ingredients:
- 2 whole grain bread slices
- ¼ avocado, mashed
- 3 tablespoons hummus
- ½ cup mixed salad greens
- ¼ cup cucumber, sliced
- ¼ cup carrot, shredded

Instructions:
1. Spread hummus on 1 bread slice and avocado mash on the other.
2. Stuff the slices with the remaining ingredients and cover with the other slice to make a sandwich.
3. Cut the sandwich in half and serve immediately.

Nutrition (Per Serving): Calories: 325Fat: 14g Carbohydrates: 40g Protein: 13g Fiber: 12g Sugar: 7gSodium: 407mg

Tip: To add more flavor, you can season the vegetables with salt and pepper and add a drizzle of hot sauce.

123. Chickpea Chile Bowl

Prep Time: 10 minutes
Cook Time: 0 minutes
Servings: 2

Ingredients:
- 1 (15 oz.) can salt-free chickpeas, rinsed
- 1 sheet nori, torn
- 1 cup carrots, shredded
- ¼ cup scallions, sliced
- 1 tablespoon sambal Oelek
- 2 teaspoons sesame seeds, toasted
- 1 teaspoon toasted sesame oil
- 1 teaspoon rice vinegar

Instructions:
1. Combine oil, vinegar, and sambal Oelek in a medium bowl.
2. Add in the remaining ingredients and toss to coat.
3. Serve immediately and enjoy.

Nutrition (Per Serving): Calories: 272Fat: 5g Carbohydrates: 41g Protein: 13g Fiber: 10g Sugar: 5gSodium: 237mg

Tip: If sambal Oelek (chile paste) is unavailable, go for red hot sauce. And if you can't find nori sheet, simply use lettuce or rice paper instead.

124. One Pot Chicken & Broccoli Pasta

Prep Time: 10 minutes
Cook Time: 10 minutes
Servings: 4

Ingredients:
- 12 oz. broccoli florets, chopped-into-bite-sized-pieces
- 8 oz. whole grain small shell pasta
- 3 garlic cloves, minced
- 2 cups water
- 2 cups salt-free chicken broth
- 2 cups cooked chicken breast, shredded
- ¾ cup whole-milk plain Greek yogurt
- ¾ cup grated Parmesan cheese, low-fat, divided
- 2 tablespoons extra-virgin olive oil
- 2 tablespoons fresh dill, chopped
- 1 ½ tablespoons Worcestershire sauce
- 1 tablespoon salt-free tomato paste
- ½ teaspoon ground pepper
- ¼ teaspoon salt

Instructions:
1. Place a high-sided skillet or large pot over high heat.
2. Add water, broth, pasta, Worcestershire, oil, tomato paste, garlic, salt and pepper and stir.
3. Bring it all to a boil and add in broccoli.
4. Stir occasionally so that the pasta doesn't stick together.
5. Cook for 7-8 minutes till the pasta is al dente, the broccoli is tender and the sauce is creamy.
6. Take it off from the heat and stir in yogurt, chicken, parmesan, and dill.
7. Dish out into serving bowls and serve immediately.

Nutrition (Per Serving): Calories: 530Fat: 18g Carbohydrates: 52g Protein: 44g Fiber: 8g Sugar: 7gSodium: 625mg

Tip: You can use leftover chicken with this recipe. And if yogurt is unavailable, you can substitute with light sour cream.

125. Chicken with Spinach Skillet

Prep Time: 10 minutes
Cook Time: 15 minutes
Servings: 4

Ingredients:
- 1 pound boneless & skinless chicken thighs, trimmed & sliced-into-bite-sized-pieces
- 4 garlic cloves, minced
- 1 medium lemon, zested & juiced
- 5 cups lightly-packed baby spinach
- ½ cup dry white wine
- 2 tablespoons extra-virgin olive oil
- 8 teaspoons Parmesan cheese, low-fat, grated
- 1 teaspoon cornstarch
- ½ teaspoon salt
- ½ teaspoon ground pepper

Instructions:
1. Place a large skillet over medium-high flame and heat oil.
2. Stir in chicken, salt and pepper.
3. Cook for 7-9 minutes until the chicken is cooked through.
4. Stir in garlic for a minute until fragrant.
5. Meanwhile, mix dry white wine and cornstarch in a measuring cup.
6. Add to the skillet with lemon juice and zest while stirring to combine.
7. Bring it to a simmer and add in a handful of spinach.
8. Cook and stir for 2 minutes until wilted.
9. Dish out into serving plates and garnish with parmesan on top.

Nutrition (Per Serving): Calories: 317Fat: 16g Carbohydrates: 11g Protein: 26g Fiber: 4g Sugar: 2gSodium: 526mg

Tip: If Parmesan cheese, low-fat, is unavailable, substitute with feta instead. To make this more filling, serve this brown rice or pasta.

Bonus Chapter 1: Mediterranean Diet Dishes

126. Chicken Salsa Verd

Prep Time: 15 minutes
Cook Time: 15 minutes
Servings: 6

Ingredients:
- 1 ½ pounds boneless & skinless chicken thighs, trimmed & cut-into-bite-sized-pieces
- 2 (15 oz.) cans salt-free rinsed pinto beans, divided
- 12 oz. (2 cups) frozen corn kernels
- 2 oz. (2 cups) spinach, chopped
- 1 medium yellow onion, chopped
- 2 large poblano peppers, chopped
- 5 garlic cloves, chopped
- 4 cups salt-free chicken stock
- 1 ½ cups prepared salsa verde
- 1 ½ cups fresh cilantro, coarsely-chopped
- 6 tablespoons sour cream
- 1 tablespoon canola oil
- ½ teaspoon salt

Instructions:
1. Place a large heavy pot over high flame and heat oil.
2. Use a masher to mash a cup of beans in a small bowl.
3. Cook chicken for 4-5 minutes, changing sides occasionally, until browned.
4. Stir in onions, poblanos, and garlic and cook for 4-5 minutes until translucent and fragrant.
5. Stir in the mashed beans, remaining beans, salsa, stock and salt.
6. Bring it to a boil and lower heat to a medium and let it simmer for 3 minutes until the chicken is cooked through.
7. Stir in cilantro, corn, and spinach and cook for a minute until wilted.
8. Ladle out into serving bowls and top with sour cream to serve.

Nutrition (Per Serving): Calories: 408Fat: 14g Carbohydrates: 41g Protein: 32g Fiber: 9g Sugar: 8gSodium: 570mg

Tip: If chicken is not available, you can use other meat varieties you like.

127. Mushroom & Kale Chickpea Pasta

Prep Time: 15 minutes
Cook Time: 15 minutes
Servings: 4

Ingredients:
- 8 oz. chickpea rotini/penne
- ¼ cup extra-virgin olive oil
- 2 large garlic cloves, sliced
- A pinch crushed red pepper
- 8 cups kale, chopped
- 8 oz. cremini mushrooms, quartered
- ½ teaspoon dried thyme
- ½ teaspoon salt
- Grated Parmesan cheese, low-fat, optional

Instructions:
1. Place a pot of water on medium-high flame and cook pasta according to the package instructions.
2. Save a cup of the pasta water and drain the rest, setting the pasta aside.
3. Place a large skillet over medium flame and heat oil.
4. Sauté garlic and red pepper for a minute.
5. Add in kale, mushrooms, thyme, and salt, stir and cook for 5 minutes until the vegetables turn tender.
6. Add in the pasta and enjoy pasta water to combine everything together easily.
7. Cook for a minute and dish out the pasta onto plates.

8. Garnish with cheese on top and serve.

Nutrition (Per Serving): Calories: 340 Fat: 18g Carbohydrates: 38g Protein: 17g Fiber: 10g Sugar: 7g Sodium: 366mg

Tip: Chickpea pasta is a good gluten-free option which is also rich in fiber, and protein. But if it is not easily available then you can also look for the whole wheat pasta to replace the chickpea pasta. To add more flavor to the recipe, you can squeeze a lemon over the pasta and add extra cheese if you like.

128. Quinoa & Chickpea Bowls

Prep Time: 20 minutes
Cook Time: 0 minutes
Servings: 4

Ingredients:
- 7 oz. jar roasted red peppers, rinsed
- 1 (15 oz.) can chickpeas, rinsed
- 1 small garlic clove, minced
- 2 cups quinoa, cooked
- 1 cup cucumber, diced
- ¼ cup red onion, finely-chopped
- ¼ cup Kalamata olives, chopped
- ¼ cup crumbled feta cheese, low-fat
- ¼ cup almonds, slivered
- 4 tablespoons extra-virgin olive oil, divided
- 2 tablespoons fresh parsley, finely-chopped
- 1 teaspoon paprika
- ½ teaspoon ground cumin
- ¼ teaspoon crushed red pepper, optional

Instructions:
1. Add 2 tablespoons of oil in mini food processor along with peppers, almonds, cumin, paprika, and crushed red pepper if desired.
2. Pulse until pretty much smooth and take out into a small bowl.
3. Meanwhile, mix quinoa, olives, red onions, and the remaining 2 tablespoons of oil in a separate medium bowl.
4. Divide the quinoa mixture among 4 serving bowls and add equal amounts of chickpea, cucumber, and the red pepper sauce.
5. Garnish with feta and parsley to serve.

Nutrition (Per Serving): Calories: 479 Fat: 25g Carbohydrates: 50g Protein: 13g Fiber: 8g Sugar: 3g Sodium: 645mg

Tip: To store this, refrigerate the sauce and the quinoa mixture in separate containers. Combine before serving only. Also, for more flavor while combining, you can sprinkle salt and pepper as per taste and squeeze lemon on top.

129. One Pot Spinach & Chicken Sausage

Prep Time: 20 minutes
Cook Time: 0 minutes
Servings: 4

Ingredients:
- 9 oz. cooked chicken sausage, thinly-cut into rounds
- 8 oz. can salt-free tomato sauce
- 6 cups whole-wheat rotini pasta, cooked
- 4 cups (½ 5 oz. box) lightly-packed baby spinach
- 1 garlic clove, minced
- 1 cup onion, diced
- ½ cup feta cheese, low-fat, finely-crumbled
- ¼ cup Kalamata olives, chopped & pitted
- ¼ cup chopped fresh basil, optional
- 2 tablespoons olive oil

Instructions:
1. Place a large straight-sided skillet over medium-high flame and heat oil.
2. Stir in onion and garlic along with chicken sausage rounds.

3. Cook for 4-6 minutes until onion starts to brown.
4. Stir in olives, tomato sauce, spinach, and pasta to cook for 3-5 minutes until bubbling and spinach is wilted.
5. Add in a tablespoon or two of water if needed to prevent the pasta from sticking.
6. Stir in feta and basil as desired and dish out to serve.

Nutrition (Per Serving): Calories: 487Fat: 20g Carbohydrates: 59g Protein: 23g Fiber: 8g Sugar: 7gSodium: 623mg

Tip: You can skip the olives if you don't like them. Also, to enhance the flavor, you can add salt as per salt.

130. Salmon Pita Bread Sandwich

Prep Time: 10 minutes
Cook Time: 0 minutes
Servings: 1

Ingredients:
- 3 oz. canned sockeye salmon, flaked & drained
- ½ (6-inch) whole wheat pita bread
- ½ cup watercress
- 2 tablespoons plain fat-free yogurt
- 2 teaspoons lemon juice
- 2 teaspoons chopped fresh dill
- ½ teaspoon prepared horseradish

Instructions:
1. Combine all the ingredients except salmon and watercress in a small bowl.
2. Lastly, stir in salmon and stuff half of the pita bread with this mixture and watercress.
3. Serve on a plate and garnish with extra chopped dill on top.

Nutrition (Per Serving): Calories: 239Fat: 7g Carbohydrates: 19g Protein: 25g Fiber: 2g Sugar: 3gSodium: 510mg

Tip: If canned salmon mentioned in the ingredients is not available, you can use fresh cooked salmon or leftovers. Or substitute it with a 5 oz. can of pink salmon.

131. Chickpea Lettuce Wraps with Tahini

Prep Time: 10 minutes
Cook Time: 0 minutes
Servings: 4

Ingredients:
- 12 large Bibb lettuce leaves
- 2 (15 oz.) cans salt-free chickpeas, rinsed
- ½ cup jarred & sliced roasted red peppers, drained
- ½ cup shallots, thinly-sliced
- ¼ cup tahini
- ¼ cup extra-virgin olive oil
- ¼ cup lemon juice, from 2 lemons
- ¼ cup toasted almonds, chopped
- 2 tablespoons fresh parsley, chopped
- 1 teaspoon lemon zest
- 1 ½ teaspoons pure maple syrup
- ¾ teaspoon kosher salt
- ½ teaspoon paprika

Instructions:
1. Take a large bowl and whisk together lemon juice, maple syrup, tahini, oil, lemon zest, paprika, salt and pepper.
2. Add in chickpeas, shallots, and peppers and toss to combine.
3. Divide about ⅓ cup of this mixture on lettuce leaves along with almonds and parsley on top.
4. Wrap the lettuce leaves around the mixture and serve in a bowl or small container.

Nutrition (Per Serving): Calories: 498Fat: 28g Carbohydrates: 44g Protein: 16g Fiber: 10g Sugar: 4gSodium: 567mg

Tip: To increase the quantity to 6 servings, simply add a third can of chickpeas and the flavor will still be perfect.

132. Mediterranean Tuna Spinach Salad

Prep Time: 10 minutes
Cook Time: 0 minutes
Servings: 1

Ingredients:
- 5 oz. can chunk light tuna in water, drained
- 1 medium orange, peeled/sliced
- 4 Kalamata olives, pitted & chopped
- 2 cups baby spinach
- 2 tablespoons parsley
- 2 tablespoons feta cheese, low-fat
- 1 ½ tablespoons tahini
- 1 ½ tablespoons water
- 1 ½ tablespoons lemon juice

Instructions:
1. Take a bowl and whisk together water, lemon juice and tahini.
2. Stir in tuna, olives, feta and parsley and combine well.
3. Place spinach on a serving plate with orange on the side.
4. Top the spinach with the tuna salad and serve immediately.

Nutrition (Per Serving): Calories: 376Fat: 21g Carbohydrates: 26g Protein: 26g Fiber: 16g Sugar: 14gSodium: 665mg

Tip: If you prefer more flavor, you can squeeze orange juice over it as well.

133. Mediterranean-Inspired Lunch Box

Prep Time: 5 minutes
Cook Time: 0 minutes
Servings: 1

Ingredients:
- 1 Persian cucumber/½ English cucumber, cut into spears
- ½ whole wheat pita bread, cut-into-4-wedges
- ¼ cup hummus
- ¼ teaspoon fresh dill, chopped
- 2 tablespoons mixed olives

Instructions:
1. Take a 4-cup divided sealable lunch box or container.
2. Arrange hummus, cucumber, pita, and olives in them.
3. If you like, you can keep the hummus and olives separate in a small foil cup before using.
4. Sprinkle dill on cucumber and refrigerate this until serving.

Nutrition (Per Serving): Calories: 194Fat: 9g Carbohydrates: 23g Protein: 8g Fiber: 7g Sugar: 4gSodium: 443mg

Tip: You can store this in the fridge for a day. You can also experiment with the recipe by adding your favorite veggies.

134. Shrimp & Feta Wrap

Prep Time: 5 minutes
Cook Time: 0 minutes
Servings: 1

Ingredients:
- 3 oz. cooked shrimp, chopped
- 1 whole wheat tortilla
- 1 scallion, sliced
- ¼ cup avocado, diced
- ¼ cup tomato, diced
- 2 tablespoons crumbled feta cheese, low-fat
- 1 tablespoon lime juice

Instructions:
1. Combine all the ingredients except tortilla in a small bowl.
2. Stuff this mixture into a tortilla and make a wrap.
3. Serve on a plate immediately!

Nutrition (Per Serving): Calories: 371Fat: 14g Carbohydrates: 34g Protein: 29g Fiber: 6g Sugar: 6gSodium: 615mg

Tip: Cooked shrimp can be found in the seafood section at the supermarket. If not available, look for a frozen version that can easily be thawed and steamed for this recipe. For more flavor, you can add sliced pickled jalapenos or use mango salsa if you like.

135. Berry & Chia Pudding

Prep Time: 8 hours 5 minutes
Cook Time: 0 minutes
Servings: 2

Ingredients:
- 1 ¾ cups fresh or frozen blackberries/raspberries/diced mango, divided
- 1 cup unsweetened almond milk/any milk
- ½ cup whole-milk plain Greek yogurt
- ¼ cup granola
- ¼ cup chia seeds
- 1 tablespoon pure maple syrup
- ¾ teaspoon vanilla extract

Instructions:
1. Add 1 ¼ cups of fruit and 1 cup milk in a blender or food processor.
2. Pulse until pureed or very smooth and scrape out into a medium bowl.
3. Mix in syrup, chia seeds, and vanilla.
4. Cover and place in the refrigerator for approximately 8 hours or for up to 3 days.
5. Take 2 bowls for serving and divide the pudding between them.
6. Layer each serving with the remaining ¼ cup of fruit, yogurt and granola on top to serve.

Nutrition (Per Serving): Calories: 343Fat: 15g Carbohydrates: 39g Protein: 14g Fiber: 15g Sugar: 18gSodium: 125mg

Tip: You can refrigerate this for up to three days. Keep this mind when making larger batches.

136. Spinach Ravioli with Artichokes

Prep Time: 5 minutes
Cook Time: 10 minutes
Servings: 4

Ingredients:
- 15 oz. can salt-free cannellini beans, rinsed
- 2 (8 oz.) packages frozen/refrigerated spinach & ricotta ravioli
- 10 oz. package frozen & quartered artichoke hearts, thawed
- ½ cup oil-packed sun-dried tomatoes, drained + save-2-tablespoons-oil
- ¼ cup fresh basil, chopped
- ¼ cup Kalamata olives, sliced
- 3 tablespoons pine nuts, toasted

Instructions:
1. Place a large pot of water over medium-high flame and bring to a boil.
2. Cook ravioli according to package instructions and drain.
3. Toss with a tablespoon of oil and place aside.
4. Meanwhile, place a large nonstick skillet over medium flame and heat the remaining tablespoon of oil.
5. Sauté and artichokes and beans for 2-3 minutes until heated through.
6. Add in the sun-dried tomatoes, ravioli, olives, pine nuts and basil.
7. Fold to combine and dish out on serving plates.

Nutrition (Per Serving): Calories: 454Fat: 19g Carbohydrates: 61g Protein: 15g Fiber: 13g Sugar: 2gSodium: 700mg

Tip: If frozen artichoke hearts are unavailable or you can find them, substitute with a 15 oz. can but make sure to drain and rinse it well.

137. One Pot Chicken Pesto Pasta

Prep Time: 15 minutes
Cook Time: 15 minutes
Servings: 6

Ingredients:
- 8 oz. whole wheat penne
- 1-pound fresh asparagus, trimmed & chopped-into-2-inch-pieces
- 7 oz. container refrigerated basil pesto
- 3 cups shredded cooked chicken breast
- ¼ cup Parmesan cheese, low-fat, grated
- 1 teaspoon salt
- ¼ teaspoon ground pepper
- Small fresh basil leaves, for garnish

Instructions:
1. Place large pot of water over medium-high flame and cook pasta according to package instructions.
2. Add asparagus in the pasta pot during the last 2 minutes of cooking time.
3. Reserve ½ cup of water and drain the rest.
4. Return the pasta to the pot along with chicken, pesto, salt and pepper.
5. Add in the reserved water, a tablespoon at a time, to get the preferred consistency and stir to combine everything.
6. Dish out the pasta and garnish with parmesan and basil to serve.

Nutrition (Per Serving): Calories: 422Fat: 18g Carbohydrates: 32g Protein: 31g Fiber: 1g Sugar: 4gSodium: 714mg

Tip: It's much more flavorful to make your own fresh pesto.

138. Easy Raspberry Muesli

Prep Time: 5 minutes
Cook Time: 0 minutes
Servings: 1

Ingredients:
- 1 cup raspberries
- ¾ cup low-fat milk
- ⅓ cup muesli

Instructions:
1. Add muesli in a bowl with raspberries.
2. Serve with milk immediately.

Nutrition (Per Serving): Calories: 288Fat: 7g Carbohydrates: 52g Protein: 13g Fiber: 13g Sugar: 21gSodium: 82mg

Tip: Don't confuse muesli with granola. Muesli is a mixture of rolled oats, dried fruit, nuts and seeds. Look for muesli that is low in added sugar.

139. Vegetables & Lentil Stew

Prep Time: 20 minutes
Cook Time: 35 minutes
Servings: 4

Ingredients:
- 2 large carrots, roughly-chopped
- 2 medium leeks, thinly-cut-into-crescents
- 1 large sweet potato, unpeeled & chopped-into-½-inch-pieces
- 3 garlic cloves, minced
- 6 cups water
- 4 cups chopped hearty greens, like kale/Swiss chard
- 1 ½ cups green/brown lentils
- 2 tablespoons extra-virgin olive oil, divided
- 2 tablespoons tomato paste
- 1 ½ teaspoons ground cumin
- 1 ¼ teaspoons white miso
- ½ teaspoon salt

Instructions:
1. Place a large Dutch oven or stockpot over medium-high flame and heat a tablespoon of oil.
2. Stir in sweet potato and cook for 6-8 minutes until lightly-browned and soft.
3. Stir in leeks and carrots and cook for 3-4 minutes until soft.
4. Stir in cumin, tomato paste, miso, garlic, and a tablespoon of oil.
5. Stir constantly for a minute until fragrant and tomato paste becomes darkened.
6. Pour in water and add lentils with salt and increase the flame to high heat to bring it to a boil.
7. Lower heat to a simmer on medium-low and cover to cook for 25 minutes until the lentils are tender.
8. Stir in the greens, cover and cook for 10 minutes more until the greens are wilted.
9. Dish out and serve immediately.

Nutrition (Per Serving): Calories: 451Fat: 8g Carbohydrates: 77g Protein: 22g Fiber: 13g Sugar: 9gSodium: 475mg

Tip: You can store this in an airtight container for a week in the fridge or freeze it for over 3 months. You can also substitute sweet potato with normal potato if you like.

140. One Pot Mediterranean Coconut Curry

Prep Time: 25 minutes
Cook Time: 20 minutes
Servings: 6

Ingredients:
- 15 oz. can salt-free chickpeas, rinsed
- 14 oz. can coconut milk
- 2 medium tomatoes, chopped
- 1 large onion, chopped
- 2 large garlic cloves, minced
- 1 medium sweet potato, cut-into-½-inch-pieces
- 1 ½ cups green beans, cut-into-1-inch-pieces
- 1 cup low-sodium vegetable broth
- ½ cup cilantro, chopped
- 2 tablespoons avocado/canola oil
- 2 tablespoons lime juice
- 1 tablespoon fresh ginger, minced
- 1 tablespoon curry powder
- 1 teaspoon cumin seeds
- 1 teaspoon mustard seeds
- ¼ teaspoon crushed red pepper
- ¾ teaspoon salt

Instructions:
1. Place a large saucepan over medium flame and heat oil.
2. Stir in cumin and mustard seeds and cook for 30 seconds to a minute until they start to pop.
3. Stir onions and cook for 3 minutes.
4. Stir in ginger, garlic, crushed red pepper, curry powder and salt.
5. Cook for a minute until fragrant.
6. Pour in coconut milk and broth, and add tomatoes, sweet potato, green beans, and chickpeas.
7. Increase heat to bring it to a boil and then lower to a simmer.
8. Cook without cover for 15 minutes while stirring frequently until the veggies become tender.
9. Take off from heat and stir in lemon juice and cilantro.
10. Dish out to serve immediately.

Nutrition (Per Serving): Calories: 312Fat: 21g Carbohydrates: 30g Protein: 7g Fiber: 8g Sugar: 9gSodium: 436mg

Tip: You can serve this rice or rice noodles to make this more fulfilling.

Bonus Chapter 2: Gluten-Free Dishes

141. Gluten-free Creamy Broccoli Salad

Prep Time: 15 minutes
Cook Time: 10 minutes
Servings: 6

Ingredients:
- 3 bacon slices
- 4 cups broccoli, chopped
- ½ cup scallions, sliced
- ½ cup extra-sharp Cheddar cheese, low-fat, shredded
- ¼ cup mayonnaise
- ¼ cup sour cream
- 4 teaspoons rice vinegar/cider vinegar
- ¼ teaspoon ground pepper

Instructions:
1. Place a large skillet over medium flame.
2. Cook bacon for 5-7 minutes until crispy and remove to a plate lined with paper towel.
3. Save a tablespoon of bacon fat and chop the bacon slices small once it's cool enough to.
4. Meanwhile, mix mayonnaise, vinegar, sour cream, reserved bacon fat, and pepper in a large bowl.
5. Add in chopped bacon, broccoli, and cheese and toss to combine.
6. Serve immediately as lunch or a side dish.

Nutrition (Per Serving): Calories: 191Fat: 17g Carbohydrates: 4g Protein: 6g Fiber: 1g Sugar: 1gSodium: 229mg

Tip: You can store this salad in the refrigerator for upto 2 days.

142. Gluten-free Warm Stuffed Potatoes

Prep Time: 15 minutes
Cook Time: 15 minutes
Servings: 4

Ingredients:
- 2 (1 ½ pounds) medium sweet potatoes
- 2 cooked & chopped bacon slices, divided
- 3 sliced scallions, divided
- ½ cup extra-sharp Cheddar cheese, low-fat, shredded
- 4 tablespoons low-fat sour cream
- ¼ teaspoon salt
- ¼ teaspoon ground pepper

Instructions:
1. Start by preheating the oven at 400 degrees F.
2. Use a fork to prick the sweet potatoes from all sides.
3. Put it in the microwave to cook for 12 minutes until soft on High.
4. Let it cool and then slice the potatoes in half lengthwise.
5. Spoon out the potato flesh onto a medium bowl, make sure the potato shells keep intact.
6. Then mix cheese, a tablespoon scallion, half bacon, salt, and pepper in the flesh.
7. Meanwhile, arrange the potato shells on a rimmed baking sheet.
8. Fill the potato shells equally with the potato mixture using a spoon.
9. Bake for 12-15 minutes until the cheese has melted and potatoes appear nicely golden-brown.
10. Remove them onto serving plates and cover each with a tablespoon of sour cream.
11. Garnish with the remaining scallion and bacon on top to serve!

Nutrition (Per Serving): Calories: 148Fat: 8g Carbohydrates: 14g Protein: 6g Fiber: 2g Sugar: 4gSodium: 338mg

Tip: Also, set the timing of the microwave according to your type because 12-15 minutes for softening potatoes are nearly not enough or in some cases, too much. Also, you can use a mild cheese if sharp is not your cup of tea.

143. Gluten-free Tomato Mussels

Prep Time: 10 minutes
Cook Time: 10 minutes
Servings: 4

Ingredients:
- 3 pounds mussels, scrubbed & debearded
- 6 ripe plum tomatoes, cored & coarsely-chopped
- 1 cup dry white wine
- 4 garlic cloves, finely chopped
- 2 teaspoons fresh parsley, chopped
- 1 teaspoon extra-virgin olive oil

Instructions:
1. Place a Dutch oven or large pot over low flame and heat oil.
2. Stir in garlic and cook for 3 from until golden and fragrant.
3. Stir in tomatoes for a minute while increasing the heat to medium.
4. Add in wine and let it come to a boil.
5. Stir in mussels, close the lid and let it steam.
6. Frequently give the pot a shake until the mussels have opened in 3-4 minutes.
7. Remove mussels that don't open and transfer the rest to a serving bowl.
8. Spoon the broth over the mussels and garnish with parsley on top.

Nutrition (Per Serving): Calories: 275Fat: 6g Carbohydrates: 15g Protein: 28g Fiber: 1g Sugar: 3gSodium: 427mg

Tip: To clean mussels, use a firm brush to scrub them under cold, running water. Use another mussel's shell to scrape the mussels clean of any barnacles. Also, before cooking, discard any mussels with cracked shells and those that don't close when tapped. Plus, pull out the beard from each of them.

144. Gluten-free Broccolini with White Beans

Prep Time: 10 minutes
Cook Time: 10 minutes
Servings: 4

Ingredients:
- 1-pound fresh broccolini, trimmed & cut-into-2- to 3-inch-pieces
- 1 (15 oz.) can dal white beans, rinsed
- 1 cup chopped leeks, white & light green parts only
- ¼ cup fresh flat-leaf parsley, chopped
- ¼ cup toasted hazelnuts, chopped
- 3 tablespoons extra-virgin olive oil, divided
- 1 ½ tablespoons lemon juice
- 1 tablespoon garlic, grated
- ½ teaspoon ground pepper
- ½ teaspoon lemon zest, grated
- ¼ teaspoon salt

Instructions:
1. Place a large cast-iron pan over medium flame and heat oil.
2. Stir in broccolini and cook for 6-8 minutes until charred and tender.
3. Remove to a plate and wipe the pan clean.
4. Lower the heat to a medium and add a tablespoon of oil in the wiped pan with garlic, leeks, and white beans.
5. Cook while stirring frequently for 4-5 minutes until golden-brown.
6. Add broccolini back to the pan, stir and cook for a minute until cooked through.
7. Remove this mixture to a plate.

8. Meanwhile, stir hazelnuts, parsley, lemon juice, zest, remaining 1 tablespoon oil, salt and pepper in a bowl.
9. Spoon this sauce over the broccolini mixture and toss to combine.
10. Serve immediately and enjoy!

Nutrition (Per Serving): Calories: 277Fat: 15g Carbohydrates: 27g Protein: 10g Fiber: 7g Sugar: 5gSodium: 216mg

Tip: Place a small dry skillet over medium-low flame. Add in chopped hazelnuts and toast for 2-4 minutes until fragrant and golden-brown while stirring continuously. Toasted nuts have the best flavor when added to salads.

145. Gluten-free Lemon & Basil Chicken

Prep Time: 10 minutes
Cook Time: 10 minutes
Servings: 4

Ingredients:
- 1 pound (4 pieces) chicken cutlets
- 3 oz. reduced-fat cream cheese, cubed
- 1 ¼ cups salt-free chicken broth
- 1 small lemon, thinly-sliced & seedless
- 2 tablespoons unsalted butter, divided
- 2 tablespoons chopped fresh basil, plus more for garnish
- 2 teaspoons garlic, minced
- ½ teaspoon salt
- ½ teaspoon ground pepper

Instructions:
1. Place a large nonstick skillet on medium flame and heat a tablespoon of butter.
2. Season chicken with salt and pepper and place in the bubbling pan.
3. Cook chicken for 3 minutes each side until cooked through and browned.
4. Remove the chicken to a plate and cover to keep warm.
5. Place the back on the stove over medium flame.
6. Add the remaining butter and swirl to coat.
7. Stir in garlic and cook for a minute until fragrant.
8. Pour broth and let it come to a boil over medium-high flame.
9. Stir in cream cheese and cook for 5 minutes until melted and thickened.
10. Stir in the lemon slices and basil and return the chicken to the pan.
11. Let it simmer over medium flame for 4 minutes until the sauce is thick and chicken is completely covered.

Nutrition (Per Serving): Calories: 236Fat: 12g Carbohydrates: 2g Protein: 29g Fiber: 1g Sugar: 5gSodium: 485mg

Tip: Serve this chicken with pasta if you want it to be filling. And you can also add some leafy green vegetables like wilted spinach.

Bonus Chapter 3: Air Fryer Dishes

146. Scallops with Lemon Herb Sauce

Prep Time: 20 minutes
Cook Time: 8 minutes
Servings: 2

Ingredients:
- 8 large (1 oz.) sea scallops, cleaned & patted dry
- ¼ cup extra-virgin olive oil
- 2 tablespoons flat-leaf parsley, finely-chopped
- 2 teaspoons capers, finely-chopped
- 1 teaspoon lemon zest, finely-grated
- ½ teaspoon garlic, finely-chopped
- ¼ teaspoon ground pepper
- ⅛ teaspoon salt
- Cooking spray, as needed

Instructions:
1. Set the air fryer at 400 degrees F and take out the basket.
2. Season scallops with salt and pepper.
3. Grease the air fryer basket with cooking spray.
4. Place the scallops inside and grease them with cooking spray too.
5. Place the basket in the air fryer.
6. Cook scallops for 6 minutes until they register an internal temperature of 120 degrees F.
7. Meanwhile, mix parsley, oil, lemon zest, garlic, and capers in a small bowl.
8. Remove the scallops to serving plates and drizzle the sauce over it to serve.

Nutrition (Per Serving): Calories: 348Fat: 30g Carbohydrates: 5g Protein: 14g Fiber: 0g Sugar: 0gSodium: 660mg

Tip: There are two kinds of scallops sold in the market: Bay scallops and sea scallops. We are using sea scallops in this recipe and recommend buying dry-packed sea scallops as they are from deep, cold ocean waters while being larger in size.

147. Sweet Orange Chicken

Prep Time: 10 minutes
Cook Time: 20 minutes
Servings: 2

Ingredients:
- 1 pound boneless & skinless chicken thighs/breasts, cut-into-1-inch-pieces
- 1 large egg
- 2 garlic cloves, minced
- Cooking spray, as needed
- ¼ cup + 1 tablespoon cornstarch, divided
- 8 tablespoons orange juice, divided
- 2 tablespoons all-purpose flour
- 1 tablespoon low-sodium soy sauce
- 1 tablespoon rice vinegar
- 1 tablespoon honey
- 1 teaspoon toasted sesame oil
- 1 teaspoon fresh ginger, grated
- ¼ teaspoon salt
- ⅛ teaspoon crushed red pepper
- Toasted sesame seeds, for garnish

Instructions:
1. Start by preheating the air fryer for 10 minutes at 400 degrees F.
2. Beat egg in a bowl and add chicken with salt, and toss to combine.
3. Take another shallow bowl and mix ¼ cup cornstarch with flour.
4. Take a chicken piece one by one, coat it with the flour mixture, shake off the excess and place them on a plate.
5. Coat the chicken pieces with cooking spray and place them in the air fryer basket.
6. Work in batches if the air fryer space is limited.

7. Cook for 8-12 minutes until crispy and the meat thermometer inserted in the thickest part of chicken reads 165° F.
8. Meanwhile, mix 2 tablespoons orange juice with remaining 1 tablespoon cornstarch in a skillet or small pan until smooth.
9. Whisk in the remaining orange juice, with sesame oil, honey, soy sauce, vinegar, garlic, ginger, and crushed red pepper.
10. Place it on medium flame and let it come to a boil.
11. Whisk occasionally for 1-2 minutes until thickened.
12. Add the cooked chicken in a medium bowl and toss with the orange juice sauce.
13. Serve with sesame seeds sprinkled on top.

Nutrition (Per Serving): Calories: 290Fat: 11g Carbohydrates: 21g Protein: 25g Fiber: 0g Sugar: 7gSodium: 418mg

Tip: To make this dish more filling, serve it with brown rice or steamed vegetables.

148. Lemony Lamb Chops

Prep Time: 10 minutes
Cook Time: 15 minutes
Servings: 2

Ingredients:
- 4 lamb loin chops
- 8 oz. baby yellow potatoes, scrubbed & halved
- 1 fennel bulb, trimmed + 2 tablespoons fronds (saved & chopped), quartered, cored & sliced
- ¼ cup Kalamata olives, chopped
- 1 tablespoon extra-virgin olive oil
- 4 teaspoons lemon zest, divided.
- ½ teaspoon salt
- ¼ teaspoon ground pepper
- Lemon wedges, for garnish

Instructions:

1. Start by preheating the air fryer for 5 minutes at 380 degrees F.
2. Coat a 6–8-quart air fryer basket with cooking spray.
3. Prepare 2 teaspoons lemon zest, salt and pepper mixture in a large bowl and use half to marinate the lamb chops.
4. Next, add potatoes, oil, and sliced fennel to the remaining lemon zest mixture and toss to coat in the bowl.
5. Place the lamb chops and vegetables in the air fryer basket in a single layer.
6. Work in batches if the air fryer space is limited.
7. Cook for 10-12 minutes, while flipping once, until a meat thermometer inserted into the middle of the lamb chop reads 145 degrees F.
8. Meanwhile, combine the remaining 2 teaspoons lemon zest, olives with fennel fronds in a bowl.
9. Remove the cooked lamb chops and vegetables to a platter and drizzle the olive mixture on top.
10. Serve with lemon wedges as you like.

Nutrition (Per Serving): Calories: 350Fat: 14g Carbohydrates: 34g Protein: 28g Fiber: 9g Sugar: 8gSodium: 906mg

Tip: You can use other types of chops with this recipe if you don't prefer lamb chops or they are unavailable.

149. Quick Tangy Zucchini

Prep Time: 10 minutes
Cook Time: 20 minutes
Servings: 4

Ingredients:
- 2 large (8oz.) zucchini, ¼-inch-thick-slices
- 2 tablespoons Parmesan cheese, low-fat, grated
- 1 tablespoon extra-virgin olive oil
- 2 teaspoons lemon juice

- ½ teaspoon salt
- ½ teaspoon dried oregano
- ¼ teaspoon garlic powder
- ¼ teaspoon onion powder
- ¼ teaspoon ground pepper
- ⅛ teaspoon crushed red pepper

Instructions:

1. Start by preheating the air fryer for 5 minutes at 400 degrees F.
2. Mix crushed red pepper, Parmesan, oil, onion powder, ground pepper, oregano, salt, and garlic powder in a medium bowl.
3. Add in zucchini slices and toss to combine.
4. Place the zucchini slices in the air fryer basket in a single layer.
5. Work in batches if the air fryer's space is limited.
6. Cook for 10-12 minutes, turning once, until crispy and golden-brown.
7. Remove to a serving plate, drizzle lemon juice on top and garnish with lemon wedges.

Nutrition (Per Serving): Calories: 64Fat: 5g Carbohydrates: 5g Protein: 2g Fiber: 1g Sugar: 3gSodium: 345mg

Tip: If your zucchini slices stick to the air fryer basket, then choose to spray a cooking spray before air frying. Also, if Parmesan cheese, low-fat, is not available, use other type of cheese for your ease.

150. Crumbed Chicken Breasts

Prep Time: 10 minutes
Cook Time: 15 minutes
Servings: 4

Ingredients:

- 4 (4 oz.) boneless & skinless chicken breasts
- ½ cup whole wheat breadcrumbs
- 1 tablespoon extra-virgin olive oil
- 2 teaspoons Dijon mustard
- ½ teaspoon salt
- ½ teaspoon paprika
- ½ teaspoon onion powder
- ½ teaspoon garlic powder
- ½ teaspoon ground pepper

Instructions:

1. Start by preheating the air fryer at 390 degrees F for 5 minutes.
2. Season the chicken breasts with salt evenly.
3. Meanwhile, mix mustard and oil in a medium bowl until combined.
4. Mix paprika, onion powder, garlic powder, breadcrumbs, and pepper in a shallow dish.
5. First dip the chicken in the oil mixture, then in the breadcrumbs to coat evenly.
6. Place the breaded chicken breasts in the air fryer basket, maintaining a ½ inch space between the pieces.
7. Work in batches if the air fryer space is limited.
8. Cook for 6 minutes each side until golden-brown and crispy, flipping once.
9. Once the meat thermometer in the thickest portion of chicken reads 165 degrees F, it's done.
10. Remove to serving plates and serve with mustard.

Nutrition (Per Serving): Calories: 227Fat: 7g Carbohydrates: 12g Protein: 27g Fiber: 2g Sugar: 0gSodium: 407mg

Tip: Serve these crispy chicken breasts with salad or your favorite dipping sauce to enhance the flavor. Also, instead of using whole wheat breadcrumbs, you can use gluten-free breadcrumbs for your personal preference.

Chapter 18: Meal Planning and Prep

You see, when you do not plan your meal, you might end up bringing the wrong ingredients home, and last-minute cooking can confuse a person between all the dos and don'ts of the diet. Meal prepping is highly recommended, especially when you are a beginner. Prepare a list of the items that are your cause of inflammation and mark them off your grocery list. Now, divide the remaining items into your routine meal in a way that could maintain the variation. Try to add more spices and herbs to the food to enjoy both the taste and good health. You can get started by following these five easy steps:

Start with simple ingredients

Use dishes that demand five to ten ingredients, except for spices and herbs. Cooking and gardening are appreciated life activities that are jammed by pain; that is why you want to keep meal preparation easy.

Eat convenient foods:

Buy low-sodium preserved beans and frozen fruits and vegetables. These are useful for emergencies for the weeks when you don't have time to go shopping. Use pre-cut fruits, salads, and vegetables for less slicing and saving time.

Cook in bulk:

Prepare the food two or three times, freeze that food, and use it for the next few days.

Meal According to Preferences:

The best thing about the anti-inflammatory diet is that it is completely flexible, and you can adjust it according to your own dietary preference. Here is what you can do:

- List the food that you enjoy the most. This list will help you organize your diet around your own choices and the principles of the anti-inflammatory diet.
- Remember your dietary requirements and limitations. If you have any dietary limitations, then choose recipes that are suitable for you.
- If you don't have a lot of time to cook, then you can cook meals that are quick to make.
- When you know your schedule, dietary requirements, and demands, you can start preparing your meals for the week. Include as many meals as you can from numerous food groups.
- When you know you are running out of the items again, make a grocery list of all the things you'll need. This will save you money and time.
- Don't stick with the same type of meals and explore other options, too; having a variety of meals on the menu keeps it interesting.
- Don't waste the leftovers. By using your leftovers, you can save your time and money. Include your leftovers in your next meal by adding more healthy seasoning or items to change the taste.
- Be inventive. Don't hold back from experimenting with new recipes and exploring new dishes by adding your favorite food items.

Meal Plan

The 31 days meal plan shared in this section will help you get started with your anti-inflammatory dietary approach, right away. It is important to note that these meal plans are created to offer 1500-2000 calories per day, so they are perfect for those who are employing portion control in their daily routine. However, based on your individual preferences, body mass index (BMI), caloric and nutritional needs you can adjust the meal plans, by adding more recipes or removing the ones that are unwanted. Feel free to use our bonus weekly meal plan template to craft your own!

Week 01

	Breakfast	Lunch	Snacks	Dinner		Dessert
Day 01	Spinach & Egg Scramble	Baked Chicken & Vegetables with Romesco Sauce	English Muffin with Tuna Salad	Chicken Salsa Verd	Strawberry Veggie Salad	Sweet & Easy Pistachio & Date Bites
Cal: 1916	296	499	349	408	296	68
Day 02	Egg & Avocado Toast	Creamy Chicken One Pot Pasta	Crispy Green Lettuce Wraps with Turkey	Mushroom & Kale Chickpea Pasta	Toasty Turmeric Cauliflower	Sweet Fig & Honey Yogurt
Cal: 1579	230	353	324	340	124	208
Day 03	Healthy Nut Butter Smoothie	Quick Beef Curry with Rice	Healthy & Creamy Pesto Chicken	Quinoa & Chickpea Bowls	Veggie Tuna Salad	Strawberry & Chocolate Yogurt Bark
Cal: 2005	402	334	324	479	432	34
Day 04	High Protein Omelet	Easy Chicken Marsala	Black Beans & Veggie Taco Bowl	One Pot Spinach & Chicken Sausage	Chicken & Mushroom Salad	Old-Fashioned Apple Crisp Dessert
Cal: 2130	339	344	435	487	384	141
Day 05	Berry Oatmeal Smoothie	Ground Beef Pasta	Healthy Goat Cheese & Arugula Sandwich	Salmon Pita Bread Sandwich	Creamy White Beans & Avocado Salad	Frozen Chocolate Banana Bites
Cal: 1774	121	582	414	239	360	58
Day 06	Chocolate & Banana Oatmeal	Quick & Crispy Chicken Thighs	Creamy Rotisserie Chicken Bowl	Chickpea Lettuce Wraps with Tahini	Chicken & Mushroom Salad	Date & Mango Energy Bites
Cal: 1812	295	332	230	498	384	73
Day 07	Salmon with Scrambled Eggs	Meatballs & Garlic-Lemon Orzo	Kale & Sun-Dried Tomatoes Snack	Mediterranean Tuna Spinach Salad	Sweet & Smoky Roasted Broccoli	Banana Flourless Chocolate Chip Muffins
Cal: 1675	205	586	326	376	104	78

Week 02

	Breakfast	Lunch	Snacks	Snacks	Dinner	Dessert
Day 08	Fried Egg & Avocado Toast	Meatballs & Garlic-Lemon Orzo	Strawberry Veggie Salad	English Muffin with Tuna Salad	Scallops with Lemon Herb Sauce	Quick Peach & Pistachio Toast
Cal: 2043	271	586	296	349	348	193
Day 09	Piña Colada-Inspired Smoothie	Sweet & Spicy Pork Kebabs	Chicken & Mushroom Salad	Crispy Green Lettuce Wraps with Turkey	Sweet Orange Chicken	Sweet Fig & Honey Yogurt
Cal: 1716	213	297	384	324	290	208
Day 10	Strawberry & Tofu Smoothie	Grilled Steak with Salad Dressing	Veggie Tuna Salad	Healthy & Creamy Pesto Chicken	Lemony Lamb Chops	Easy Watermelon Sherbet
Cal: 1818	171	409	432	324	350	132
Day 11	High Protein Omelet	Salmon Piccata with Sauce	Chicken & Mushroom Salad	Black Beans & Veggie Taco Bowl	Quick Tangy Zucchini	Sweet & Easy Pistachio & Date Bites
Cal: 1602	339	312	384	435	64	68
Day 12	Berry Oatmeal Smoothie	Quick Crispy Salmon	Creamy White Beans & Avocado Salad	Healthy Goat Cheese & Arugula Sandwich	Crumbed Chicken Breasts	Sweet Fig & Honey Yogurt
Cal: 1607	121	277	360	414	227	208
Day 13	Chocolate & Banana Oatmeal	Burrata Pasta with Cherry Tomatoes	Chicken & Mushroom Salad	Creamy Rotisserie Chicken Bowl	White Bean Pasta Soup	Strawberry & Chocolate Yogurt Bark
Cal: 1718	295	498	384	230	277	34
Day 14	Salmon with Scrambled Eggs	Ground Beef Pasta	Creamy White Beans & Avocado Salad	Kale & Sun-Dried Tomatoes Snack	Veggie Minestrone Soup	Old-Fashioned Apple Crisp Dessert
Cal: 1846	205	582	360	326	232	141

Week 03

	Breakfast	Lunch	Snacks	Dinner		Dessert
Day 15	Spinach & Egg Scramble	Crusted Sweet Scallops	English Muffin with Tuna Salad	Broccoli with Tofu Stir Fry	Strawberry Veggie Salad	Sweet & Easy Pistachio & Date Bites
Cal: 1547	296	281	349	257	296	68
Day 16	Egg & Avocado Toast	Grilled Steak with Salad Dressing	Crispy Green Lettuce Wraps with Turkey	Chicken-Style Seitan Stir Fry	Toasty Turmeric Cauliflower	Sweet Fig & Honey Yogurt
Cal: 1648	230	409	324	353	124	208
Day 17	Healthy Nut Butter Smoothie	One Pot Shrimp with Spinach	Healthy & Creamy Pesto Chicken	Chinese green beans stir fry	Veggie Tuna Salad	Strawberry & Chocolate Yogurt Bark
Cal: 1579	402	226	324	161	432	34
Day 18	High Protein Omelet	One Pot Shrimp & Broccoli	Black Beans & Veggie Taco Bowl	Creamy Brussels Sprouts with Fettuccine	Chicken & Mushroom Salad	Frozen Chocolate Banana Bites
Cal: 1814	339	214	435	384	384	58
Day 19	Berry Oatmeal Smoothie	Mediterranean-Style Cod with Tomatoes	Healthy Goat Cheese & Arugula Sandwich	Goat Cheese & Beet Pasta	Creamy White Beans & Avocado Salad	Date & Mango Energy Bites
Cal: 1593	121	151	414	474	360	73
Day 20	Chocolate & Banana Oatmeal	Crispy Pan-Fried White Bass	Creamy Rotisserie Chicken Bowl	Chickpea Salad with Cranberry & Walnut	Chicken & Mushroom Salad	Banana Flourless Chocolate Chip Muffins
Cal: 1633	295	250	230	396	384	78
Day 21	Salmon with Scrambled Eggs	Hearty Shrimp & Fish Stew	Kale & Sun-Dried Tomatoes Snack	One Pot Spinach & Chicken Sausage	Sweet & Smoky Roasted Broccoli	Sweet Fig & Honey Yogurt
Cal: 1657	205	327	326	487	104	208

Week 04 and extra days

	Breakfast	Lunch		Snacks	Dinner	Dessert
Day 22	Fried Egg & Avocado Toast	Burrata Pasta with Cherry Tomatoes	Strawberry Veggie Salad	English Muffin with Tuna Salad	Baked Chicken & Vegetables with Romesco Sauce	Quick Peach & Pistachio Toast
Cal: 2065	230	498	296	349	499	193
Day 23	Healthy Nut Butter Smoothie	One Pot Shrimp with Spinach	Toasty Turmeric Cauliflower	Healthy & Creamy Pesto Chicken	Quinoa & Chickpea Bowls	Strawberry & Chocolate Yogurt Bark
Cal: 1589	402	226	124	324	479	34
Day 24	Salmon with Scrambled Eggs	Garlic Pea Shoots Stir Fry	Veggie Tuna Salad	Black Beans & Veggie Taco Bowl	Quick Beef Curry with Rice	Easy Watermelon Sherbet
Cal: 1688	205	150	432	435	334	132
Day 25	High Protein Omelet	Spicy Broccoli Stir Fry	Chicken & Mushroom Salad	Healthy & Creamy Pesto Chicken	Easy Chicken Marsala	Quick Peach & Pistachio Toast
Cal: 1843	339	259	384	324	344	193
Day 26	Berry Oatmeal Smoothie	Peanut Butter Broccoli Stir Fry	Creamy White Beans & Avocado Salad	Healthy Goat Cheese & Arugula Sandwich	Ground Beef Pasta	Sweet & Easy Pistachio & Date Bites
Cal: 1699	121	154	360	414	582	68
Day 27	Chocolate & Banana Oatmeal	Lemon Asparagus Stir Fry	Chicken & Mushroom Salad	Creamy Rotisserie Chicken Bowl	Quick & Crispy Chicken Thighs	Sweet Fig & Honey Yogurt
Cal: 1561	295	112	384	230	332	208
Day 28	Salmon with Scrambled Eggs	Broccoli with Tofu Stir Fry	Strawberry Veggie Salad	Kale & Sun-Dried Tomatoes Snack	Meatballs & Garlic-Lemon Orzo	Strawberry & Chocolate Yogurt Bark
Cal: 1704	205	257	296	326	586	34
Day 29	Spinach & Egg Scramble	Baked Chicken & Vegetables with Romesco Sauce	Toasty Turmeric Cauliflower	English Muffin with Tuna Salad	Chicken Salsa Verd	Sweet & Easy Pistachio & Date Bites
Cal: 1744	296	499	124	349	408	68
Day 30	Egg & Avocado Toast	Creamy Chicken One Pot Pasta	Veggie Tuna Salad	Crispy Green Lettuce Wraps with Turkey	Mushroom & Kale Chickpea Pasta	Sweet Fig & Honey Yogurt
Cal: 1887	230	353	432	324	340	208

Conclusion

With the positive mindset, progress approach and gradual changes, anyone can harness the benefits of a diet. The important thing is to keep the process consistent. An anti-inflammatory diet is effective in coping with all forms of inflammation; its results are free from any side effects and are long-lasting. This is the reason that even medical specialists are now prescribing the masses to opt for this diet and be free from the harm of inflammation. I have offered you this cookbook to help you incorporate this dietary approach into your life with convenience. With its collection of 150 recipes, you will have lots of options to not only cook for yourself but also for your family. So ahead, give my 30 meals plan a try and give back your valuable feedback. Your constructive criticism is an important of my book writing process, and it really helps me improve my writing game.

But wait, Hold on!

There are more **BONUSES** coming your way:

BONUS 1 - 30 Days Meal Plan Grocery List: Kickstart your health journey with a ready-made grocery list tailored for our meal plan. No guesswork, just grab and go!

BONUS 2 - Foods to Eat & Avoid Cards: A quick cheat sheet to keep your meals anti-inflammatory friendly. Know what to embrace and what to avoid at a glance.

BONUS 3 - Grocery List: A template featuring the most common healthy foods. Quickly jot down what you need for your recipes and take it shopping—effortless and efficient.

BONUS 4 - Recipe Card: Discover a new favorite? Note it down and make it a heart-healthy classic in your kitchen.

BONUS 5 - Weekly Meal Plan Template: Flex your culinary creativity with a customizable template.

The bonuses are 100% FREE

You only need to provide your name and email; no additional information is required.

Unlock your exclusive bonuses NOW by scanning the QR code!

Note from the Author:

Hello, Health Hero!

You've aced another recipe, and we're thrilled you're with us. But before you go, know this: your words matter.

Two Birds, One Stone

We're indie authors on a budget; your review means a lot to us and keeps us going. Plus, it lights the way for others fighting health issues. It's a win-win!

Time's Ticking—Speak Up!

The faster you review, the quicker we help more people. Health waits for no one.

Thanks a lot for staying with me!

Grace Garner

Measurement Conversion Table

Weight conversion tables

Pounds (lbs.)	Ounces (oz)	Grams (g)
1	16	453.6
2	32	907.2
3	48	1360.8
4	64	1814.4
5	80	2268.0

Kilograms (kg)	Pounds (lbs.)	Ounces (oz)	Grams (g)
0.5	1.1	17.6	500
1	2.2	35.3	1000
1.5	3.3	52.9	1500
2	4.4	70.5	2000
2.5	5.5	88.2	2500
3	6.6	105.8	3000

Ounces (oz)	Grams (g)	Tablespoons (tbsp)	Teaspoons (tsp)
0.5	14.2	1	3
1	28.4	2	6
1.5	42.5	3	9
2	56.7	4	12
2.5	70.9	5	15
3	85.0	6	18
3.5	99.2	7	21
4	113.4	8	24
4.5	127.6	9	27
5	141.7	10	30

Liquid Conversion Table

Measurement	Metric	US Customary	Imperial
Teaspoon (tsp)	5 ml	1/6 fl oz	1/6 fl oz
Tablespoon (tbsp)	15 ml	1/2 fl oz	1/2 fl oz
Fluid Ounce (fl oz)	30 ml	1 fl oz	1.04 fl oz
Cup (c)	240 ml	8 fl oz	9.61 fl oz
Pint (pt)	473 ml	16 fl oz	19.22 fl oz
Quart (qt)	946 ml	32 fl oz	38.43 fl oz
Liter (l)	1000 ml	33.814 fl oz	35.195 fl oz
Gallon (gal)	3.785 l	128 fl oz	153.72 fl oz

Recipe Index (Alphabetical order)

Asparagus & Cauliflower Gnocchi, 74
Bacon with Brussels Sprouts, 33
Baked Chicken & Vegetables with Romesco Sauce, 30
Banana Flourless Chocolate Chip Muffins, 64
Berry & Chia Pudding, 87
Berry Oatmeal Smoothie, 17
Black Beans & Veggie Taco Bowl, 57
Broccoli with Tofu Stir Fry, 49
Brown Rice & Black Beans Bowl, 75
Burrata Pasta with Cherry Tomatoes, 45
Buttered & Seared Scallops, 70
Butternut Squash Soup with Halloumi, 72
Calamari with Fresh Herbs Salad, 43
Chicken & Mushroom Salad, 27
Chicken & Strawberry Poppy Seed Salad, 72
Chicken Ginger & Garlic Soup, 24
Chicken Salsa Verd, 83
Chicken with Spinach Skillet, 82
Chicken-Style Seitan Stir Fry, 50
Chickpea & Pomegranate Salad, 29
Chickpea Chile Bowl, 81
Chickpea Lettuce Wraps with Tahini, 85
Chickpea Salad with Cranberry & Walnut, 53
Chinese green beans stir fry, 51
Chocolate & Banana Oatmeal, 18
Creamy Brussels Sprouts with Fettuccine, 51
Creamy Chicken One Pot Pasta, 30
Creamy Cucumber Salad Sandwich, 60
Creamy Kale Salad, 28
Creamy Rotisserie Chicken Bowl, 58
Creamy White Beans & Avocado Salad, 28
Crispy Green Lettuce Wraps with Turkey, 56
Crispy Pan-Fried White Bass, 41
Crumbed Chicken Breasts, 96
Crusted Sweet Scallops, 38
Date & Mango Energy Bites, 63
Easy & Creamy Chipotle Sauce, 67
Easy Chicken Marsala, 31
Easy Pesto Ravioli, 70
Easy Raspberry Muesli, 89
Easy Sauteed Spinach, 28
Easy Watermelon Sherbet, 65
Easy White Wine Sauce, 67

Edamame & Beets Salad, 76
Egg & Avocado Toast, 16
English Muffin with Tuna Salad, 56
Falafel & Tzatziki Tabbouleh Bowls, 60
Fish Fillets with Lemon-Dill Sauce, 43
Fried Egg & Avocado Toast, 19
Frozen Chocolate Banana Bites, 63
Garlic Pea Shoots Stir Fry, 47
Gluten Free Broccolini with White Beans, 92
Gluten Free Creamy Broccoli Salad, 91
Gluten Free Lemon & Basil Chicken, 93
Gluten Free Tomato Mussels, 92
Gluten Free Warm Stuffed Potatoes, 91
Goat Cheese & Beet Pasta, 52
Grilled Steak with Salad Dressing, 35
Ground Beef Pasta, 32
Healthy & Creamy Pesto Chicken, 57
Healthy Goat Cheese & Arugula Sandwich, 58
Healthy Kale & Banana Smoothie, 76
Healthy Nut Butter Smoothie, 17
Hearty Lentil Soup with Saffron, 20
Hearty Shrimp & Fish Stew, 41
High Protein Omelet, 17
Homemade Garlic Aioli, 66
Homemade Rosemary & Red Wine Marinade, 69
Indian Paneer Saag, 77
Instant Ramen Noodles With Soft-Boiled Egg, 59
Italian Olive Dressing, 66
Kale & Sun-Dried Tomatoes Snack, 59
Lemon & Garlic Vinaigrette, 68
Lemon Asparagus Stir Fry, 48
Lemon Fiddleheads Stir Fry, 48
Lemony Lamb Chops, 95
Meatballs & Garlic-Lemon Orzo, 33
Mediterranean Tuna Spinach Salad, 86
Mediterranean-Inspired Lunch Box, 86
Mediterranean-Style Cod with Tomatoes, 40
Moo-Shu Chinese Style Vegetables, 46
Mushroom & Kale Chickpea Pasta, 83
Old-Fashioned Apple Crisp Dessert, 62
One Pot Chicken & Broccoli Pasta, 81
One Pot Chicken Pesto Pasta, 88
One Pot Mediterranean Coconut Curry, 90

One Pot Shrimp & Broccoli, 40
One Pot Shrimp with Spinach, 39
One Pot Spinach & Chicken Sausage, 84
Orange Tofu with Chipotle, 79
Panko & Pistachio Crusted Halibut, 39
Peanut Butter Broccoli Stir Fry, 48
Piña Colada-Inspired Smoothie, 19
Pineapple & Tofu Stir Fry, 53
Quick & Crispy Chicken Thighs, 32
Quick & Easy Cucumber Pickles, 68
Quick & Fresh Pineapple Ice Cream, 65
Quick Barley Bean Soup, 24
Quick Beef Curry with Rice, 31
Quick Black Bean Quesadillas, 71
Quick Crispy Salmon, 36
Quick Peach & Pistachio Toast, 64
Quick Tangy Zucchini, 95
Quick Vegetarian Chili, 79
Quinoa & Chickpea Bowls, 84
Roasted Garlic Parmesan Cream Sauce, 69
Salmon & Peppercorn Sauce, 44
Salmon Piccata with Sauce, 36
Salmon Pita Bread Sandwich, 85
Salmon with Scrambled Eggs, 18
Scallops with Lemon Herb Sauce, 94
Seasoned Grilled Red Snapper Fish, 37
Shrimp & Feta Wrap, 87
Simple Baked Fish Fillets, 42
Simple Blackened Catfish, 37
Slow Cooker Veggie Chili Soup, 23
Spicy Broccoli Stir Fry, 47
Spinach & Egg Scramble, 16
Spinach & Walnut Pesto, 66

Spinach Ravioli with Artichokes, 88
Steamed Green Beans, 75
Strawberry & Chocolate Yogurt Bark, 62
Strawberry & Tofu Smoothie, 19
Strawberry Veggie Salad, 26
Stuffed Avocado with Salmon, 75
Stuffed Potatoes & Salsa, 71
Stuffed Sweet Potatoes, 74
Sweet & Easy Pistachio & Date Bites, 61
Sweet & Smoky Roasted Broccoli, 27
Sweet & Spicy Pork Kebabs, 34
Sweet Fig & Honey Yogurt, 61
Sweet Orange Chicken, 94
Sweet Potato & Quinoa Chili, 78
Sweet Tart Balsamic Marinade, 68
Teriyaki Edamame Stir Fry, 73
Tex-Mex Black Beans & Fajita, 73
Toasted Shishito Peppers, 45
Toasted Zucchini Stir Fry, 49
Toasty Turmeric Cauliflower, 26
Tuna with Chickpea Salad, 77
Vegetable Soup for Slow Cooker, 21
Vegetable Soup with Parmesan, 23
Vegetable Soup with Pesto, 20
Vegetables & Hummus Sandwich, 80
Vegetables & Lentil Stew, 89
Vegetarian Fried Rice, 80
Veggie Minestrone Soup, 22
Veggie Tuna Salad, 26
Veggie-Packed Tofu Soup, 25
White Bean Pasta Soup, 21
Whole Grain Quinoa & Pea Salad, 29

Made in United States
North Haven, CT
24 February 2024

49168545R00059